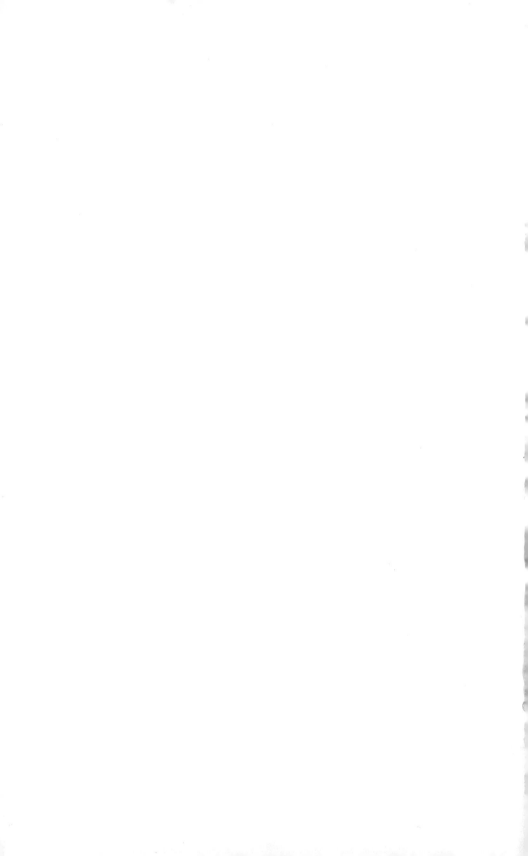

Individualized Dementia Care

Joanne Rader, RN, MN, is a Clinical Research Fellow at the Benedictine Institute for Long Term Care and Associate Professor at the Oregon Health Sciences University School of Nursing. She holds a master's degree in nursing from Oregon Health Sciences University. She was Project Director for a three-year grant from the Robert Wood Johnson Foundation (1991–1993) to develop a model for changing practice related to the use of physical restraints and psychoactive medications in nursing in Oregon homes. Ms. Rader has had numerous articles published addressing behavioral symptoms of the cognitively impaired such as wandering, aggression and on individualizing care for persons with dementia.

Elizabeth Tornquist, MA, teaches scientific writing in the School of Nursing and School of Public Health, University of North Carolina at Chapel Hill. She has a master's degree in English from the University of Chicago and is an editor and former journalist. Ms. Tornquist has authored numerous articles on scientific and technical writing and has edited a series of volumes on the utilization of research in nursing practice.

INDIVIDUALIZED DEMENTIA CARE

CREATIVE, COMPASSIONATE APPROACHES

Joanne Rader, RN, MN, FAAN

Elizabeth M. Tornquist, MA, Editor

Benedictine Institute for Long-Term Care

Springer Publishing Company

Springer Publishing Company, Inc.
536 Broadway
New York, NY 10012-3955

Cover design by Tom Yabut
Production Editor: Pam Lankas

95 96 97 98 99 / 5 4 3 2 1

Library of Congress Cataloging-in-Publication Data

Individualized dementia care: creative, compassionate approaches / Joanne Rader, Elizabeth M. Tornquist, editors.
     p.   cm.
  Includes bibliographical references and index.
  ISBN 0-8261-8730-7
  1. Alzheimer's disease—Nursing. 2. Dementia—Nursing.
  3. Alzheimer's disease—Patients—Long-term care. 4. Dementia—Patients—Long-term care. I. Rader, Joanne. II. Tornquist, Elizabeth   M., 1933– .
     [DNLM: 1. Dementia—nursing. 2. Long-Term Care—trends.
  3. Long—Term Care—methods. 4. Patient Care Planning.
  5. Professional—Patient Relations. 6. Caregivers.
  WM 220 C737   1995]
  RC523.C66 1995
  362.1'9683—dc20
  DNLM/DLC
  for Library of Congress   94-45714
                                                                            CIP

Printed in the United States of America

This book is dedicated to my nursing mentor,
Sr. Marilyn Schwab, my Mother, Marjorie Faber,
who first taught me about caring, and to my husband
Tom, and sons Josh, Jim, and Andy, who continue as my teachers.

CONTENTS

vii

Part IV   Appendices

FOREWORD

Increasing discontent with the nature of long-term care in our country has led to a call for a paradigm shift—away from a hospital-like, paternalistic, dehumanizing model toward one that is resident-centered, individualized, and holistic in nature. The routine use of physical restraints with frail older residents has come to symbolize all that is "wrong" with the old model: A focus on tasks rather than the person; the importance of a smoothly functioning unit rather than on support of the normal routines of everyday life; and the primacy of eradication, cure, and control of symptoms over attention to the meaning of behavior.

Nightingale's 1859 principle, "What nursing has to do . . . is to put the patient in the best condition for nature to act" (p. 75), is clearly violated by the use of restraints, which have well-established morbidity and mortality outcomes. Restraint used to manage what is perceived by staff as "challenging behavior" leads, thus, to poorer quality of care. Further, such practice contributes to poorer quality of life by disrupting the trusting relationship between resident and helper so necessary for understanding. In contrast, good geriatric care embraces goals of independent functioning, including rehabilitation and restoration, reasonable risk-taking for normal everyday life, and respect for the dignity and individuality of the older person. Older adults, like most people, function best in environments in which they feel safe and secure and that are homelike, individualized, and normalized. In such environments, a true community of caring that supports reasonable risk-taking, respects personal dignity, and enhances quality of life can evolve.

In this book, Rader has clearly demonstrated how this subtle but essential paradigm shift can occur, and she has described the positive outcomes for residents, families, and staff when it does. Even the title captures the excitement of discovery and creativity that this kind of nursing represents. With the realization that resident behavior may be something different from what it at first seems, caregivers are challenged and assisted to take on roles of magician, detective, carpenter, and jester to *reframe* resident behavior, *search* for its meaning, *customize* a response to meet individual needs, and approach situations with a *sense of humor*. The author recognizes that the kind of caring that can result from this type of approach is so different from the status quo that she refers to it as "magic".

What Rader espouses is actually much more than "magic." She presents methods to assure that such care is rigorously planned, systematic, objective, and based on empirical as well as experiential evidence. Although acknowledging the importance of organizational commitment to the new way of caring, Rader recognizes that staff will need assistance in refining skills for observing, assessing, decision making, and developing strategies to meet residents' needs within a reasonably safe environment. The concept that behavior should be viewed as a symptom to investigate rather than a problem to be "solved" or "controlled," whether by physical restraints or inappropriate psychoactive drugs, is often new to caregivers. Our research has documented that although staff can benefit from formal education about these new concepts of care, resident-centered consultation together with education is most efficacious in changing behavior (Evans, et al. 1994).

As Collopy, Boyle, and Jennings (1991) have stated, "Caring constitutes the fabric of the person's life" (p. 9). This books's reaffirmation of caring—the essence of nursing—is refreshing. Rader challenges the reader to "return to basics," beginning first with a focus on recreating caring, loving relationships and getting to "know the patient as a person," rather than relying on a "standard-ized care plan." Further, nurses are empowered to think more critically about customary ways of caring, including use of re-straints, management of incontinence, and bathing and feeding routines. As noted, many of the methods currently in use have no empirical basis, are supported by myths and continued merely out of habit, and, like restraint use, often have iatrogenic outcomes (Evans & Strumpf, 1990).

Nationally, the effort to improve the quality of long-term care by reducing restraint use and enhancing the dignity and personal choices of residents has been facilitated through the decade-long efforts of consumer-advocacy groups, dedicated clinicians, gerontologic researchers, policymakers, and legislators (Strumpf & Evans, 1992). Although the standard of nursing home care is rap-idly changing, mere removal of restraints will not automatically result in good quality, humane care. A major transformation in attitudes and the paradigm of long-term care is essential to this evolution. It may be timely to reflect that, with regard to elimina-tion of routine restraint in psychiatric care, we were almost there 100 years ago (Strumpf & Tomes, 1993). Although those efforts at reform were not entirely successful, a new opportunity is upon us to modify dramatically and radically the way we care for another at-risk population—the frail and demented elderly. This book goes a long way toward assuring success this time.

Lois K. Evans, RN, DNSc, FAAN
Neville E. Strumpf, RN, PhD, FAAN

REFERENCES

Collopy, B., Boyle, P., & Jennings, B. (1991). New directions in nursing home ethics. *Hastings Center Report, 21*(2, Special Suppl.), 1–16.

Evans, L. K., & Strumpf, N. E. (1990). Myths about elder restraint. *Image, 22*(2), 124–128.

Evans, L., Strumpf, N., Taylor, L., Jacobsen, B., Capezuti, E., & Maislin, G. (1994). A clinical trial to reduce restraints in nursing homes [Abstract], *Gerontologist, 34*(6, Special Issue).

Nightingale, F. (1859). *Notes on nursing*. Philadelphia: Lippincott.

Strumpf, N. E., & Evans, L. K. (1992). Alternatives to physical restraints: Editorial. *Journal of Gerontological Nursing, 18*(11), 4.

Strumpf, N. E., & Tomes, N. (1993). Restraining the troublesome patient: An historical perspective on a contemporary debate. *Nursing History Review, 1*(1), 3–24.

ACKNOWLEDGMENTS

The first author wishes to thank the Robert Wood Johnson Foundation (Grant 17311) for funding the Oregon Restraint Reduction Project, from which this book evolved, and my friends and colleagues on the project, Joyce Semradek, Darlene McKenzie, and Mary Lavelle, for their support and invaluable insights. In addition, I am grateful to Shirley Saries and Cindy Hannum for their commitment to making new and better ways of caring for elderly persons, described in this book, a reality in Oregon. I also would like to thank Luanne Richey and Gloria Garcia for their gracious assistance and patience in the preparation of the manuscript.

I am deeply grateful to the staff, residents, and families of the Benedictine Nursing Center for having the courage, creativity, and commitment to develop and implement the concepts of caring presented in this book.

For their encouragement, advice and assistance in reading and editing versions of the manuscript, I wish to thank Vicki Schmall, Julia Brown, Carter Williams, Sarah Green Burger, and Janet Tulloch.

The work of Lis Wagner and Ulla Turremark, colleagues in Denmark and Sweden, continues to inspire me and I am thankful for the time and energy they spent showing me what a compassionate, caring model looks like in practice.

To my friends and nursing colleagues, Lucia Gamroth, Joy Smith, Bev Hoeffer, Lynda Crandall, Ann Marie Monahan, Lori Linton-Nelson, and Maggie Donius I am ever grateful for their ears, advice, insights, and friendship.

JOANNE RADER

CONTRIBUTORS

Lynda Crandall, RN, C., GNP, is a Gerontological Nurse Practitioner on the Outreach Team of the Geropsychiatric Treatment Program at Oregon State Hospital. She has worked for 20 years in geriatric mental health providing direct care in the hospital and nursing home settings. In addition, she provides consultation and training to a variety of settings and frequently presents at conferences in the Northwest and throughout Oregon. Ms. Crandall has authored training manuals and several chapters in a text on nursing management of the elderly.

Maggie Donius, RN, MN, is a Gerontology Clinical Nurse Specialist at the Benedictine Nursing Center in Mt. Angel, Oregon. She is an assistant professor at the Oregon Health Sciences University School of Nursing and in that capacity is serving as an Associate Director of Professional Development for the Oregon Geriatric Education Center. She is interested in clinical isues common to frail older people and enjoys very much being a nurse in a nursing home.

Deborah A. Jones, PT, is a physical therapist with a special interest in wheelchair positioning and mobility for the elderly in long-term care. She is a national educator regarding principles and key elements required to seat the elderly in the long-term care setting. She is a clinical consultant for the Benedictine Institute for Long Term Care in Mt. Angel, Oregon and a clinician at the King City Rehabilitation and Living Center in Tigard, Oregon.

William Simonson, Pharm D, is an Associate Professor of Pharmacy Practice with the Oregon State University College of Pharmacy in Portland, Oregon. Dr. Simonson has published many articles on the use and misuse of medications and the elderly and is the author of two books, *Medications & The Elderly: A Guide for Promoting Proper Care* and *Consultant*

Pharmacy Practice. He presently serves as a member of the editorial board of *Drug Regimen Review: A Process Guide for Pharmacists* and is a member of the United States Pharmacopeia Advisory panel on Geriatrics. He is a member of the Oregon Board of Examiners of Nursing Home Administration and is actively involved in clinical research involving elderly patients.

Kurt Smidt-Jernstrom, MDiv, MA, is the interfaith chaplain at the Benedictine Nursing Center in Mt. Angel, Oregon. He is also a pastoral counselor with Kaiser Permanente Hospice in Portland. Mr. Smidt-Jernstrom is a consultant in ethics and is active in denomination responsibilities (United Church of Christ).

Melinda Sullivan, RN, MS, is a Psychiatric Nurse Practitioner and faculty member at Oregon Health Sciences University in Portland, Oregon. Her clinical experience has a strong emphasis on geriatric nursing. Currently she is in clinical practice at the Portland Veteran's Administration Medical Center.

Doris Weaver, MA, Ed, is a gerontological consultant and counselor specializing in care of persons with dementia. She served as coordinator of Aging Services and Coordinator consultant for the Alzheimer's Resource Center, Good Samaritan Outreach Services, Puyallup, Washington. In addition, she coordinated the National Council on Aging Intergenerational Service Project at Oregon State University and has been in private practice. She is well-known in the northwest as a dynamic speaker, innovator, and motivator in the area of care for the elderly individual and their family.

PART I

AN INQUIRY APPROACH
TO CAREGIVING

Chapter 1

MOVING AWAY FROM THE HOSPITAL MODEL TO AN INDIVIDUALIZED RESIDENT-CENTERED MODEL

Joanne Rader

The traditional model of nursing home care grew out of a hospital model. Recently, we have become painfully aware of the many shortcomings of that model and the ways in which it has created problems for staff and, more important, has limited the choice, dignity, and normalcy of the individuals who reside in nursing homes. Rising health care costs and the "graying" of America compel providers, consumers, and regulators to work together to create new models of care. Although new models such as in-home care, assisted living, and foster care are emerging, it seems clear that the nursing home will still be necessary for many individuals, and it appears that a large proportion of those people will be suffering from some form of dementia.

The hospital model in no way fits the needs of patients with dementia, and in fact, it creates many problems that are manifested in difficult behavioral symptoms; these in turn impair residents' ability to function at their highest possible level and create stress and burnout in nursing home staff. Observations of a number of special care units suggest that when the total environment, including organizational, physical, and psychosocial aspects, is

3

structured to meet the needs of a specific population, rather than asking the population to adapt to the environment, there is a dramatic improvement in the quality of life of residents and a decrease in the "problem behaviors" with which staff must cope (Mace, 1993).

However, although the number of special care units is growing, no one model has proved to be "ideal" (OTA Report, 1992). In addition, as the number of nursing home residents who are suffering from the later stages of dementia increases, whole facilities will need to embrace the concepts that have emerged from successful special care units.

The question becomes, how do we meet the needs of demented nursing home residents safely and efficiently yet honor the rights of individuals? With hospital models, it seems impossible. However, with new models, the answers appear with startling simplicity and clarity.

One factor that has been critical in bringing about change is the federal regulations (OBRA, or Omnibus Budget Reconciliation Act of 1987) that went into effect in October 1990. OBRA established new practice standards for addressing "problematic" behavioral symptoms and, in particular, for using physical restraints and psychoactive medications. The Health Care Financing Administration's Interpretive Guidelines and Resident Assessment Protocols (RAPS) Related to the Use of Physical Restraints and Psychoactive Medications provide very specific information to providers and regulators concerning the use of these interventions. OBRA regulations emphasize the importance of supporting dignity, freedom, choice, and quality of life for nursing home residents. As a result, long-term care facilities are dramatically changing the way they deal with behaviors labeled "problematic."

In the past, little information and few guidelines were available to caregivers on how to deal with problematic behavioral symptoms. Ten years ago almost no studies had been done, and the literature included only a few anecdotal reports on dealing with such problems. The tools caregivers had to work with were physical restraints, psychoactive medications, and reality orientation. The use of restraints was considered necessary for several reasons:

- To prevent residents from wandering away from a facility and becoming lost or injured
- To prevent confused individuals from interfering with necessary treatments
- To maintain posture and provide support for those with weakened musculature
- To control disruptive behaviors, such as aggression and restlessness thought to be dangerous to the resident or others
- To prevent falls

We have now learned that these old approaches have only limited value. There is overwhelming evidence that physical restraints have negative effects. Indeed, there is now considerable evidence that people fall in spite of restraints. Further, the data indicate that while the number of falls may increase with decreased restraint use, the number of serious injuries related to falling does not increase. New, practical theories and approaches have emerged. We have learned that it is important to listen to residents and their families, to carefully observe resident behavior, and to consider whether a resident's behavior may be expressing an unmet need. We have learned to ask the "why" of behavior and the "who" of the individual.

It is critical for all those involved in long-term care to grasp the true intent of the OBRA reforms. Providers need to be aware that these regulations seek to shift the focus of enforcement from "paper compliance" to helping residents attain their highest mental, physical, and psychosocial well-being. The new regulations indicate that care must be individualized, physical restraints should be rarely, if ever, used, and psychoactive medications should be used much less frequently and more appropriately. The Interpretive Guidelines and survey process are two tools for implementing this new philosophy of care. The Surveyor's Interpretive Guidelines provide a framework for implementing and evaluating the changes required but not a road map. There are many other tools as well.

Together, the new forces have created a window of opportunity within the long-term care health system to put into practice a new way of truly "caring" for individuals. This is a crucial time to push caregiving systems to change and to embrace a more fitting, appropriate, and humanistic approach to care.

There are many factors that make this transition difficult: fear of litigation; the high staff turnover rates in many facilities; regulatory and sanction pressures; lack of experience; and lack of clear standards to guide providers, regulators, advocates, and consumers in implementing this new philosophy of care.

This volume is designed to articulate the new attitude and new approach to examining behavioral symptoms; to increase caregivers' knowledge and skill in understanding behavioral symptoms; to assist providers, regulators, and consumers in identifying appropriate care practices and standards related to behavioral symptoms; and to describe the components of a thoughtful process for determining individual care needs. The book can serve as a guide to understanding, preventing, and redirecting difficult behavior and thereby help caregivers to dramatically reduce or eliminate physical restraints and to reduce—and use more appropriately—psychoactive medications.

A major premise of the volume is that most "problematic" behavioral symptoms can be prevented if caregivers first develop a relationship with each resident and know the resident well enough to answer the question, "Who is this person?" (C. Williams, personal communication, 1993). The next step is to look at behaviors not as the resident's problem but as a symptom that expresses an unmet need. Knowledge gained from the relationship with the resident can guide the search for the unmet need.

Building a relationship with the resident is crucial to understanding his/her behaviors. Most behavioral symptoms occur in people with dementia who cannot tell us directly that something is wrong. However, behavioral symptoms are cues that something is wrong; they express an unmet need. If we have ongoing relationships with residents, we can recognize changes in behavior and thus have a basis for identifying underlying problems. For example, a woman caring for her mother at home knew that one behavior her mother manifested as part of her dementia was repetitive spelling of words. When her mother suddenly began misspelling words, the daughter knew that something was wrong and began investigating possible underlying causes. In fact, the mother had developed a urinary tract infection, and the first indication of the problem was the behavior change—misspelling words. Without the daughter's knowledge and questioning, the problem probably would not have been identified. Her mother's behavior might have escalated into agitation and perhaps combativeness because of the discomfort from the urinary tract infection.

Developing a relationship can be rewarding for both the caregiver and the resident. It requires that the caregiver use good communication skills; observe the resident; gather information about the resident's past interests, behaviors, daily schedules, and coping patterns; and learn what was and is important to the resident.

A relationship develops over time, as the staff learns "who this person is" and mutual trust is built. The more the staff knows, the easier it is to intervene effectively when behavioral symptoms occur.

Various interactions require different degrees of relationship. For example, a person doing an assessment or consultation may meet with the resident only one or two times, but it is important to develop good rapport to enable the resident to function at his or her maximum level during the assessment.

In contrast, staff in long-term care settings have daily opportunities over extended periods, often years, to get to know residents very well. The quality of the relationship between staff and resident often determines the behavior of both.

Knowledge about a resident's prior behavioral symptoms and their meaning can be acquired through observations and through talking to family, friends, and past caregivers. Questions that are pertinent to ask include these:

- To whom does the resident best relate?
- What kind of relationships have sustained the resident through life?
- Do some relationships seem threatening or show evidence of old wounds?
- Does the resident seem to work better with certain staff members?

It is impossible to individualize care unless you have a relationship with the resident. To individualize care requires learning about the individual's life history, assessing the individual's current strengths and needs, developing plans with resident and/or family input, and designing care around the resident's wishes and needs—not facility, staff, or family needs. A sense of what interventions might be useful will emerge from knowledge of the person's history, desires, coping style, supports, deficits, strengths, needs, and reactions to others.

Individualized care will often look and sound different from traditional care. It requires moving from generalized to resident-centered, specific approaches. For example, the presence of chin hairs on Mrs. Smith cannot be assumed to mean that her dignity is not being respected or that she is not being cared for properly. It may be an indication of her personal preference. And if Mr. Reels, a cognitively impaired resident, only recognizes the word "poop" to describe his need to defecate, then it is appropriate for staff to word their questions accordingly: "Do you have to poop?" This is not infantalizing or degrading but skillful individualized care based on a particular resident's needs. To provide another illustration, Mrs. Scharf, who was dying with metastatic cancer, found any movement very painful and requested that she no longer be turned or positioned routinely. The staff should honor the request and evaluate the pain control program. The usual "turn every 2 hours" routine would not be appropriate, and concerns about skin breakdown should be less important than her need for comfort.

Most of the emotional content of our communication comes in facial expressions, body posture, and tone of voice, rather than words. Individuals with dementia have impaired speech and language skills, but they are exquisitely attuned to the moods and attitudes of those around them. For example, a staff member may be greeted on first meeting as if she were a long-lost friend if her approach (verbal and nonverbal) conveys a kind, interested, calm openness. Good communicators observe others' responses and alter their behavior to facilitate the relationship.

For residents with severe dementia, who may be bedfast and incontinent at night, being awakened every 2 hours for continence care and positioning may be very disruptive and frightening, resulting in resistive and combative behaviors. Several of those on the night staff have reported that one technique they tried when they knew a particular resident might be combative was to "sneak" in to do the care in hopes of not fully awakening the resident. Another technique was to go in and fully awaken the resident, making sure there were enough staff present to hold onto the resident's arms and perhaps legs to prevent hitting, scratching, and kicking. Neither of these approaches seems to have worked well for either the resident or the staff. Allowing the resident to sleep makes more sense. The purpose of the 2-hour routine is to maintain good skin integrity and positioning and to prevent odor. However, these goals can often be accomplished in other ways, such as allowing the resident to awaken naturally before providing care.

Because the every-2-hour ritual has become an accepted, expected practice, staff personnel often do not perceive that they have care choices and that alternatives are acceptable. A question frequently asked by nursing home staff is "What will the surveyors say?" The answer is that with the new OBRA focus on outcomes, if an alternate plan based on a thorough, documented assessment is developed, with input from resident and family, there should be no problem with individualized approaches that vary from standard routines.

REFERENCES

Mace, N. L. (1993). Observations of dementia specific care around the world. *American Journal of Alzheimer's Care and Related Disorders and Research, 1*(3), 1–8.

Office of Technology Assessment, U.S. Congress. (1992). Special care units for people with Alzheimer's and other dementias: Consumer education, research, regulatory and reimbursement issues. Washington, DC: U.S. Government Printing Office.

Chapter 2

EXPLORING CONTROL AND AUTONOMY ISSUES

Joanne Rader

CONTROL AND AUTONOMY

The system of health care that places the physician or other care provider in the role of primary decision maker is changing. The movement toward increased patient autonomy is strong in this country, as evidenced by the growing recognition that personal decision making plays a role in maintaining a sense of well-being, the move toward honoring nursing home residents' rights, the use of advance directives and durable power of attorney for health care, ombudsmen programs, and the new survey process. The word *autonomy* etymologically means self-rule. In practice it has come to convey a multitude of "connected and overlapping notions: liberty of thought and action, the inviolability of the self, the freedom of individuals to choose from among a plurality of beliefs and values, the right to be singular, idiosyncratic, even eccentric, to live on one's own plural recognizance" (Collopy, 1994). In the nursing home setting, individuals, particularly those with dementia, come face to face with others (staff) who also are choosing and acting. "Thus, thinking about autonomy leads us to reflect on questions of power, on others who can support or suppress autonomy, bring it resources or restraints" (Collopy, 1994).

Most care providers were educated and still practice in a system that is paternalistic and controlling. The underlying assumption is that caregivers know best and need to protect care receivers from making poor judgments.

Initially, giving control back to the care receiver often feels like a noncaring act because it goes against the training and mind-set that many caregivers have had about what constitutes good care. Therefore, it is useful to rethink what is "good care." The current changes in the use of physical restraints provide a good model for this.

In the United States, over several decades, physical restraints evolved as the intervention of choice for managing falls, interference with treatment, agitation, and wandering (Evans & Strumpf, 1989). This standard, though scientifically untested and based purely on consensus, became accepted practice in most U.S. health care settings. To not restrain patients perceived to be at risk was viewed as negligence by caregivers, administrators, some families, regulators, and, at times, the legal system. The caregiver was expected to control residents' behavior so as to prevent them from harming themselves.

Individuals both with and without dementia do not tolerate well attempts to control their behaviors by the use of restraints. Fortunately, the standard has now changed. We are aware that restraints have few benefits and overwhelmingly negative consequences. The negative consequences of restraint use and the consequences of immobility include withdrawal/humiliation/depression; regressive behavior; resignation; resistance/anger/agitation; increased cognitive impairment; decreased appetite; dehydration; changes in body chemistry, metabolism, and blood volume; cardiac stress; stress response (increased corticosteriods); EEG changes; and decreased function of the blood-brain barrier. Numerous deaths related to restraint use have been documented (Miles & Irvine, 1992). Complications of immobilization also include circulatory obstruction/edema/pressure ulcer, muscle atrophy/contracture, bone demineralization, respiratory problems, infections, increased incontinence, and orthostatic hypotension.

Positive consequences of restraint use documented in the literature are limited to recommendations for restraint use, but research evidence demonstrating their usefulness does not exist.

We must learn to recognize that residents have the right to choose to take risks. The story of Mr. Torrence illustrates the changes in caregiver thinking that need to occur if residents are to have choice and autonomy. Mr. Torrence had had a stroke, but he wished to continue independently going to the toilet in spite of several falls and some bumps and bruises, though no serious injuries. Discussing this, a staff member said, "My blood pressure can't take worrying about his falling under my care." Her statement was meant as an expression of caring about the resident's well-being. What the caregiver failed to recognize was that she was putting her own emotional well-being above the well-being of the resident, who was quite able to understand the possible consequences of his choice. This particular resident would even try to hide from staff as a way to avoid restraints and maintain his freedom to go to the toilet on his own.

It was necessary for the staff to reframe their role in this situation—from preventing all falls to supporting the resident's desire for independence by minimizing the risks of injury. The staff needed to understand that a fall or even an injury is not negligence if a thoughtful process has been used to assess the risks and benefits of various approaches, if the parties involved recognize risk taking as an essential part of life and self-respect, if a negotiated safety plan has been developed with the resident and/or family, if the plan is carried through, and if the plan is reevaluated as necessary.

We can learn a great deal about control and autonomy from the recent drastic changes in restraint use in long-term care settings. First, the examination of restraint use illustrates that much of what we consider to be practice based on scientific evidence is really based only on consensus and beliefs about what is best for others. Second, it shows how often we choose interventions for others "in their best interest" that we would never want for ourselves. Finally, it illustrates how limited the vision of caregivers can become when they allow their care to turn into a series of tasks and rituals, rather than an assessment of individual needs.

Once caregivers in long-term care absorb the full meaning of the changes in restraint use, a whole new vista of options opens up in other areas of care. Take, for example, bathing. Many facilities have policies and procedures related to routine bathing of residents, that is, a bath or shower (often the mode is chosen by the caregiver without consulting the resident or family) at a particular time or on a particular day of the week. Little effort is made to determine the resident's preferences and past patterns. It is not uncommon to see a nursing home resident taken kicking and screaming into the shower room. We generally treat persons with dementia as if they no longer have the right to say no.

Looking at the bath or shower from the perspective of a resident with dementia, we see a different picture. A person she does not recognize enters the room, removes her from her bed, begins taking off her clothes, all against her verbal and often physical protests. Her calls for help go unheeded; others ignore her pleas as she is moved down a very public hall cold and naked except for a thin sheet that barely covers her private parts. Her verbal cries for help are greeted only with casual smiles or ignoring. She enters a cold, foreign-looking room, the sheet is removed, and again, against her wishes and protests, she is sprayed with often too cold water or too hot water while this stranger touches her private parts. In any other context, that behavior would be considered an assault. Is it any wonder that the person with confusion becomes verbally and physically assaultive in response?

Instead of interpreting their resistive and combative behaviors as an indication that they can no longer tolerate this method of maintaining hygiene and we need to individualize the process, we label the resistance a behavior problem and justify forcing the residents to endure the process, sometimes even medicating them for "resistance to care." However, if we learn from our experience in developing alternatives to restraints, we will begin looking for other ways to maintain hygiene that may or may not include a routine shower or bath. Many people maintain quite adequate cleanliness by sponge baths at the sink or bed baths. A towel bath procedure (see Table 2.1), in which the resident is covered with a warm, moist towel during the bed bath (Calgon-Vestal Laboratories, 1975) is a comfortable, pleasant time-saving alternative for some residents. Again, when you look at the individual and her needs, freed from the constraints of control, parentalism and routines, solutions will emerge.

Table 2.1   The Towel Bath: A Gentle Bed Bath Method for Nursing Home Residents

Equipment
- 2 bath blankets
- 1 large plastic bag containing:
  1 large (6'6" × 3') light-weight towel (fan folded)
  1 standard bath towel
  2 washcloths
- 2-quart plastic pitcher filled with bath temperature water (approximately 105°F), to which you have added:
  1 ounce of no-rinse soap (such as Septa-Soft, manufactured by Calgon-Vestal)

Preparing the Resident

Explain the bath. Make the room quiet or play soft music. Dim the lights if this calms the resident. Assure privacy. Wash hands. If necessary work one bath blanket under the resident, to protect the linen and provide warmth. Undress the resident, keeping him/her covered with bed linen or the second bath blanket. You may also protect covering linen by folding it at the end of the bed.

Preparing the Bath

Pour the soapy water into the plastic bag, and work the solution into the towels and washcloths until they are uniformly damp but not soggy. If necessary, wring out excess solution through the open end of the bag into the sink. Twist the top of the bag closed to retain heat. Take the plastic bag containing the warm towels and washcloths to the bedside.

Bathing the Resident

Expose the resident's shoulders and upper chest, and immediately cover the area with the warm, moist large towel. Then gently and gradually uncover the resident while simultaneously unfolding the wet towel to recover the resident. Start washing at whatever part of the body is least distressing to the resident. For example, start at the feet and cleanse the body in an upward direction by massaging gently through the towel. Wash the backs of the legs by bending the person's knee and going underneath. As you move upward, roll the towel upward and cover the person with the bath blanket. After bathing the

(continued)

Table 2.1   *Continued*

trunk, bathe the face, neck, and ears with the end of the towel at the neck area. You may also hand one of the washcloths to the resident and encourage him/her to wash his/her own face. Turn the resident to one side and place smaller warm towel from plastic bag on back, washing in a similar manner, while warming the resident's front with the bath blanket. No rinsing or drying is required. Use a washcloth from the plastic bag to provide perineal care. Gloves should be worn when washing perineal and rectal areas.

After the Bath

If desired, have the resident remain unclothed and covered with the bath blanket and bed linen, dressing at a later time. A dry cotton bath blanket (warmed if possible) placed next to the skin and tucked close, provides comfort and warmth. Place used linen back into plastic bag, tie the bag and place in a hamper.

Adapted with permission from "Towel-Bath—Totman Technique." St. Louis: Calgon-Vestal Laboratories, 1975.

"PROBLEM" LANGUAGE

The language we use in discussing "problem behaviors" often reflects the need for caregiver control. We talk about behavior problems, behavior modification, and behavior management. These terms imply that the problem rests solely with the resident and it is the caregiver's responsibility to "control" the behavior of others—a difficult task at best.

We need to develop a new way of discussing behaviors, one that is more neutral and resident-centered. One useful way to describe behaviors is to refer to difficult behaviors as behavioral symptoms; recognize that the causes of behavior often exist outside the resident—for example, in an unsupportive environment; describe behavioral symptoms as reflections of an unmet or unidentified need and/or a response to stressors in the environment (Burger, 1992); and describe plans and approaches in terms of resident needs, supports, and strengths and what staff can do to meet needs—not in terms of behavior management and modification.

One of the first questions we need to ask is "Whose problem is it?" Many resident behaviors are problems for others, not the resident. For example, one nurse resident care manager has observed that many psychoactive drugs are given for behaviors that are personality traits rather than behavior problems. All individuals have characteristics that are irritating and problematic for others, but once we become adults, it is not generally accepted that others should decide that our irritating traits need to be altered and develop and implement a plan (which may include medications) to change them without our approval or involvement.

The following examples illustrate "problems" that, using a new way of looking at behaviors, are no longer considered to belong to the resident:

Mildred and Fred, two confused residents, greatly enjoy each other's company and like to hold hands, kiss, and occasionally share the same bed. The family of one insisted that the behavior be stopped. The problem was the family's, and they needed support and education; the staff did not, however, need to develop an elaborate plan for keeping the residents separate: it was not the residents' problem.

Mr. Eldridge, a bright, active resident suffering from cerebral palsy, had been in an institution for many years. He was frequently frustrated by the constraints of the institution and the controlling attitudes of some staff members. At times this frustration took the form of swearing at staff. The language did no physical harm and is a commonly used coping mechanism that the resident chose as an outlet for frustration. It was offensive to some of the staff at times. Whose problem is it?

REFERENCES

Burger, S. (1992). Eliminating inappropriate use of chemical restraints [Special section]. *Quality Care Advocate, 7*, i–iv.

Collopy, B. (1995). Power, paternalism and the ambiguities of autonomy. In L. Gamroth, J. Semradek, & E. Tornquist (Eds.), *Enhancing autonomy in Long-Term Care: Concepts and Strategies.* New York: Springer Publishing Company.

Evans, L., & Strumpf, N. (1989). Tying down the elderly: A review of the literature on physical restraints. *Journal of American Geriatrics Society*, 37(1), 65–74.

Miles, S. H., & Irvine, P. (1992). Deaths caused by physical restraints. *The Gerontologist*, 32(6), 762–766

Towel Bath—Totman Technique. (1975). St. Louis: Calgon Vestal Laboratories.

Chapter 3

THE PROBLEM-SOLVING PROCESS

Joanne Rader

When we observe behaviors in another that seem dangerous, disruptive, unacceptable, or "wrong," our response is generally to try to get the individual to change the behavior. However, this approach is nearly always ineffective. It neglects to find out what is causing the behavioral symptoms. If someone had hot skin, you would want to know why. Is it dehydration or infection? The treatment for the two problems is very different. This is also the case with behavioral symptoms: you need to know the cause before you can successfully respond. It is crucial to be open and take an inquiring approach to problems, always searching for alternative solutions.

Many residents in nursing homes lack the physical, cognitive, and coping resources to change their behaviors. So it becomes the responsibility of caregivers to determine the cause and discover what can be altered to reduce or eliminate disruptive resident behaviors.

Identifying residents' unmet needs, conducting a physical assessment, consulting the physician, choosing the appropriate medical and behavioral intervention(s), and evaluating the response can be a complex task. It is helpful to view the process of understanding behaviors and solving problems as a sequence of roles that staff

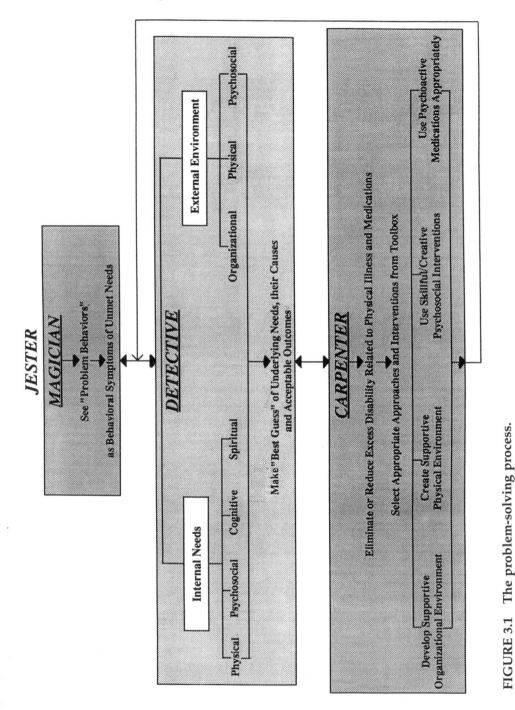

FIGURE 3.1   The problem-solving process.

take on (see Figure 3.1). These are the roles of magician, detective, carpenter, and jester.

THE MAGICIAN

The first role that staff must assume is that of the magician. The magician's job is to step into the resident's shoes and turn "problem behaviors" into behavioral symptoms of unmet needs or reactions to stress in the eyes of everyone involved in the individual's care.

What we know about magic is that much of it is an illusion. What seems impossible becomes possible if you have the knowledge and skill and know the "tricks." For example, the Wizard of Oz's "magic" was simply to provide a symbol to the tin man, lion, and scarecrow for what they thought they lacked. That symbol allowed them to bring out in themselves traits that already existed. Skillful, caring staff members have the ability to bring out the best in even the most difficult residents and situations. Skillful supervisors and administrators also know how to do this with their staff.

An important task of the magician is to "become" the resident and experience the world through the resident's eyes, ears, and feelings. The world of the nursing home can be experienced from the resident's perspective in many ways. In a concrete sense, it may mean that staff sit in the residents' wheelchairs or lie in their beds. For example, when a resident was having difficulty sleeping and staying in bed at night, the old approach might have been to use restraints and medications. However, an aide used a magician's trick. She lay down in the resident's bed, and there she discovered that the light from the hall shone directly into her eyes. Removing the light bulb resolved this woman's "agitation" and "sleep disturbance" (Burger, 1992).

Restlessness and poor posture of residents in wheelchairs may be due to discomfort or poor support. Asking the resident what he is experiencing physically in the chair or having a staff member sit in the chair or wheelchair can often uncover underlying causes of restlessness that are easily corrected.

In a more abstract sense, "becoming" the resident means using your knowledge about the resident's past history, skills, and ability to cope with the current situation. It is a form of empathy. Emotionally experiencing the world as the resident does may be difficult. The best source of information about his experiences is the resident himself. However, residents are often unable to directly provide the information. The family or significant others can help. However, remember, this information is filtered through their view of the resident's needs and wishes and cannot completely represent the resident's perspective. Other individuals who are involved with the resident are also important. It is especially important to ask questions of those working closest to the resident, for example, the certified nursing assistants. Volunteers and housekeeping staff also often have meaningful conversations with residents and insight into their needs.

"Listen" to nonverbal messages. Even when residents are unable to provide verbal information, they usually give strong clues to their feelings by nonverbal cues. For example, a person with a nasogastric tube who attempts to pull it out every time she has the chance may not be able to verbalize what it means to discontinue the tube, but the behavior is a clear message that the tube is a great burden to her.

Residents who appear vegetative or "nonresponsive" are in fact able to communicate many things, such as discomfort or burden. As you get to know the resident, the eyes (the "windows to the soul") will communicate; caregivers learn to "read" the message and alter care based on that observation. Having a consistent long-term relationship with the resident is especially helpful in this.

THE DETECTIVE

The detective's job is to uncover clues that lead to identifying underlying unmet needs. A good detective uses several techniques for discovering clues to unmet needs. These include using the senses, following intuition and hunches, and asking questions. First and foremost, staff must look for undetected or inadequately treated acute and chronic illnesses and medication side effects and reactions. Frail older persons are at high risk for confusion and behavioral symptoms resulting from poorly treated or unidentified medical conditions and medication side effects.

The next step in the detective's job is to look inside the individual to evaluate his personal strengths and needs. Assessing a resident's internal needs requires knowing a great deal about who this person is and was. A good detective seeks information from the resident even if he is confused. What does the resident think is wrong or is needed? A good detective also talks to family members who are aware of the person's past needs and coping styles and asks questions of those who work closely with the resident, such as the certified nursing assistant. It is also important for the detective to ask others about their hunches and intuitions, as well as honoring his own. Questions might include these:

- How would you describe the person's behavior?
- What do you think is causing the behavior?
- What seems to make it worse?
- What happens just before the behavior occurs?
- What happens after the behavior occurs?
- How often does the behavior occur?
- What staff behaviors provide comfort to the resident?
- What types of activities seem to decrease the behavioral symptoms and provide pleasure for the resident?
- How did the resident cope with problems earlier in his life?
- Does time of day, rest, noise, pain, or eating affect the behaviors?
- How does the person's behavior affect other residents and vice versa?

Your detective work may yield a clear unmet need and solution. However, if elements of mystery remain, you will need to make your "best guess" about what is the underlying need or cause for the behavior. Unmet needs can emanate from within the resident and/or stressors in the external environment (see chapter 5).

It is also part of the detective's job to evaluate whether the correct underlying cause has been identified and whether the interventions selected are effective.

THE CARPENTER

Once you have identified the probable cause of behavioral symptoms or the underlying need, it is time to move into the role of the carpenter. The carpenter's job is to reduce any illness or medication-induced excess disability and select appropriate approaches and interventions for building an individualized plan of care.

After the carpenter sees that all physical illnesses and symptoms are treated, if appropriate, and rules out current medications as a cause of behavioral symptoms, she moves to four major categories of tools—or interventions—to use in trying to meet a resident's needs. These are developing a supportive organizational structure; creating a supportive physical environment; using creative, skillful psychosocial interventions; and using psychoactive medications appropriately.

A good carpenter expects to have many assistants or teammates, has a wide variety of tools to choose from, learns how to use the tools correctly, keeps up to date, keeps tools in good repair, creates a healthy work environment, and knows how to choose the right tools for each job.

The resources that help the carpenter add and update skills are important. Resources may include reference books; consultants; methods to evaluate progress toward goals, identify successes, and obtain feedback; and useful devices and equipment. The types of tools the carpenter uses for a particular resident depend on the results of the magician's and detective's work. If the cause of the behavioral symptom is clearly identified, then the task of choosing interventions is simple, as illustrated by the examples below.

Mrs. Moseley, who had Alzheimer's disease, yelled frequently without any apparent provocation. After looking at all the internal needs of Mrs. Moseley and the external environment, the consensus of the team was that she yelled because of arthritic pain exacerbated by transfers and manipulation of joints during care. The intervention of choice was to routinely and adequately treat the arthritic pain with medication and handle her joints more gently during care and positioning. The need expressed by yelling was for pain relief and tender care.

Mr. Johnson, a cognitively intact male resident, suddenly began asking women to go to bed with him. This had not happened previously in the nursing home, nor had it occurred in his long years as a widower in a small town. A review of medications indicated that he was now taking antiparkinson medications, which can increase libido as a side effect. In light of this unwanted, embarrassing side effect, the appropriate intervention was to reevaluate Mr. Johnson's medication.

When the cause of the behavioral symptom is unclear, the team must make a "best guess" about which intervention would be most useful. It does not matter if the first "best guess" is incorrect. If your interventions are unsuccessful, you will simply need to rethink the situation. Be sure to allow enough time to pass to truly judge whether or not the intervention is successful.

If, given enough time, the first best guess does not result in the desired outcome and the behavioral symptom continues, then you return to the role of the detective and make another best guess about the underlying cause of the behavior. It may be that the carpenter selected the wrong tool, or maybe the detective's best guess about the need was not correct. A good detective is always alert for signs that something is amiss, picking up clues to unmet needs and noting signs of diminution, persistence, or recurrence of the need. No good detective lets a mystery remain unsolved. He continues to gather facts that will shed light on the problem.

Mr. Richey, a patient with dementia, illustrates this process. Mr. Richey wandered every day at 3:30 p.m. It was difficult to know why this happened, and he had no family to ask. The staff planned for Mr. Richey to be in a small group with others at this time, but he always tried to leave. A year later, a neighbor happened to drop by to visit him, and the staff discovered that Mr. Richey had worked as a janitor on the evening shift. Thereafter, they gave him a broom and he practiced his trade instead of wandering.

THE JESTER

Humor is an important element in coping, but it is often over-looked. Everyone is aware that long-term care can be full of tragedy and loss. It is less well known that it is also full of rewards, joy, and humor. Because problem solving can be a frustrating process at times, humor is necessary. The jester lightens the load, enhances creativity, energizes, releases tension, and promotes relationships. Remember to bring the sense of humor and fun of the jester into the roles of the magician, detective, and carpenter. To illustrate, one nurse reported that she found that many demented residents were more willing to take their medication when distracted by the red clown nose she wore when she offered medications. Another used a hand puppet to get a withdrawn, depressed resident to talk. Another had her pet bird perched on her shoulder when she made rounds. Each was implementing the jester role to improve care.

When solutions seem unclear or unsuccessful, taking a deep breath and looking for humorous elements is often energizing. A bit of lightness and mirth can ease the load for all and often will free people to think of new ideas and solutions. Appealing to the resident's sense of humor is also important.

REFERENCE

Burger, S. (1992). Eliminating inappropriate use of chemical restraints [Special section]. *Quality Care Advocate, 7,* i–iv.

PART II

REFRAMING BEHAVIOR

Chapter 4

ASSESSING THE RESIDENT'S NEEDS

Melinda Sullivan, Kurt Smidt-Jernstrom, and Joanne Rader

Individuals have a number of aspects to their lives that collectively make up their overall sense of well-being. These areas include the physical, psychosocial, cognitive, and spiritual. If a person experiences a problem or unmet need in any of these areas, it may be manifested as a behavioral symptom.

This chapter describes a systematic approach to assessing the internal needs of the long-term care resident. The approach involves obtaining a history of the resident, reviewing physical status, evaluating mental status, conducting a psychosocial assessment, and assessing spiritual needs.

Assessment of older adults is a challenging task because of their potential for multiple problems, including acute or chronic physical illness, acute or chronic psychological illness, multiple losses, and polypharmacy. The "detective" of the previous chapter tries to uncover clues that will help improve the quality of life for the long-term care resident.

Understanding, preventing, and redirecting problematic behavioral symptoms for persons with dementia requires that staff become familiar with basic concepts such as excess disability and catastrophic reactions. Both of these concepts give the staff a way of reframing behaviors to view them as symptoms of unmet needs rather than problems that rest solely with the resident to change or fix.

Excess disability exists when a person's functional incapacity is greater than is warranted by actual impairment (Brody, Kleban, Lawton, & Silverman, 1971). Excess disability may be caused by unrecognized, untreated, or inadequately treated medical conditions or by the emotional, psychological, and environmental components of illness. Excess disability often results in behavioral symptoms. We can eliminate or reduce the excess disability by having medical conditions evaluated and treated, evaluating medications carefully for side effects, using medications appropriately, modifying the physical environment, and interacting with residents in more skillful ways.

Mrs. Snyder, a newly admitted resident suffering from dementia, suddenly started striking at staff during her morning care, a new behavior for her. In talking to the family, the staff discovered that she had been receiving a nonsteroidal antiinflammatory drug for her arthritis at home in the morning, but the diagnosis and medication order were not part of her admission information. The nurse called to get the order, and the medication was given routinely; Mrs. Snyder's combative behavior immediately ceased.

The care provider, with the pharmacist, should also look carefully at medications as potential causes of difficulties. The job is to reduce or eliminate any medication that may be causing the symptoms. For example, Dr. Toomey, a retired professor of mathematics, suffered from Parkinson's disease and mild dementia. Recently, her motor symptoms had worsened, and her medications were increased. She had some improvement in her ability to function, but she began having fits of rage in which she would throw objects at the staff and other residents. In addition, she would use the phone in her room to dial 911 and tell the operator that the staff was trying to kill her and she needed to get off the bedpan. A review of her medication changes indicated that she was probably experiencing delirium related to the increase in antiparkinson medications. Several medication regimens were tried. However, only on a lower dose were the rage episodes and delusions about the staff diminished. At this level of medication she was not able to regain her previous functional status. A conference, including input from a pharmacist and physician, was held to discuss these issues, and Dr. Toomey decided that the medication's behavioral side effects were more burdensome than the loss of function; therefore, the current medication regimen remained unchanged.

The resident with dementia may sometimes experience catastrophic reactions—sudden emotional outbursts and feelings of terror related to being overwhelmed, distressed, or confused by situations or failing (Mace, 1984). The specific behaviors of the resident during this catastrophic reaction will vary from occasion to occasion and from resident to resident. They may include sudden verbal and physical outbursts, stubbornness, abrupt tears, combativeness, and/or fear.

The "detective" can help solve the mystery of what is causing the behavioral symptoms by examining the behavior to see if it is a symptom of an illness, such as Alzheimer's disease, and if so, whether its frequency and intensity can be diminished by reducing excess disability. A sudden increase in catastrophic reactions is often an early indication of an undetected medical problem. For example, staff detectives of one facility learned that the first sign manifested by Helen when she was getting a urinary tract infection was sudden weepiness when a staff member approached her to do care activities. When this behavior was observed, staff would begin increasing Helen's fluid intake to prevent or minimize the infection so that antibiotics could be avoided and Helen could experience greater comfort.

HISTORY OF THE RESIDENT

Many persons in long-term care have conditions that prevent directly obtaining a thorough history. However, reviewing the chart and talking with the family or friends will provide a framework. A good history includes identifying data, a description of the current situation, the resident's concerns, and a personal history. Most identifying data can be found in the chart. It includes the resident's name, date and place of birth, sex, marital status, and name of the closest relative.

Information about the current situation can be obtained from members of the care team, family members, and the resident. It should yield a chronological summary of the development of the behavioral symptoms. It is important to obtain the perspective of the resident and quote this verbatim. For persons with dementia, asking the family to identify and communicate stressors, soothers, and signs is helpful. Stressors are things that the person finds upsetting, and soothers are things that calm or comfort the person (Beedle, 1991). Signs are what you watch for that indicate the person is becoming upset or uneasy.

Information about personal history should be sought that will help to understand the present situation. Pertinent information may include education, past employment, past ways of coping with stress, and any traumatic experiences—recent and throughout the life cycle.

The medical history should include available information about illnesses, accidents (including recent falls), hospitalizations, and surgeries, in chronological order. In addition, note past and present medications and any drug or alcohol abuse, and review laboratory data. Other areas to explore include these:

- Allergies
- Medication effects (has there been a recent change in medications?)
- Medication side effects
- Habits such as tobacco, caffeine, alcohol, and diet
- Past psychiatric history, both self and family
- Sexual concerns

THE RESIDENT'S PHYSICAL STATUS

A wide variety of treatable conditions can cause changes in a resident's behavior and mental status. The first step in assessment is to identify and treat any of these (see Figure 4.1). To enumerate these pathologies is to catalog almost every illness, intoxicant, or metabolic disturbance known to humankind.

Metabolic Disorders	Infections	Post-operative States	Intoxication
hypoxia related to anemia hypercarbia hypoglycemia hyperosmolarity dehydration ionic imbalance (sodium, potassium, calcium, magnesium, phosphorus) liver disease (hepatic encephalopathy) kidney disease (uremic encephalopathy)	urinary tract pneumonia septicemia malaria typhoid fever meningitis encephalitis	metabolic imbalance anesthetic effects infection	alcohol sedatives anticholinergics opiates stimulants L-dopa Digoxin heavy metals carbon monoxide

Overdose or Adverse Reactions	Neurological Diseases	Nutrition	Sensory Deprivation
alcohol sedatives/hypnotics (i.e., benzodiazepines) steroids antipsychotics narcotics polypharmacy	epilepsy, unobserved seizures head trauma, subdural hema- toma tumors of the brain	malnutrition decreased Thiamine (B1) vitamin deficiency	sight hearing touch

FIGURE 4.1 Treatable medical conditions that can cause behavioral symptoms.

It is a challenge to uncover the cause of acute mental or behavioral change in a resident with many medical problems. In the past, mental or behavioral changes in older persons were viewed as the norm. However, misdiagnosis is likely to occur when the mental or behavioral change becomes the primary focus of intervention rather than the underlying pathology. We now look for underlying and reversible causes.

The primary goal should be to treat the underlying illness. It is important to be persistent in the search for a cause and to communicate skillfully with the physician, giving accurate information and suggestions of possible causes. Successful treatment often depends on nursing staff's ability to clearly and convincingly communicate the assessment to the physician.

THE RESIDENT'S MENTAL STATUS

An assessment of the resident's mental status is the basis for ruling out various diagnoses that could account for the resident's problems. To determine a resident's mental status, it is important to conduct a comprehensive mental status examination. This is designed to systematically gather subjective and objective data from observations and clinical tests, to obtain a clear and accurate picture of the resident's mental status.

There are five basic sources of information for a mental status examination:

1. The resident's "case history" (i.e., the residents account)
2. The resident's family and friends
3. Medical data
4. The clinician's informal observations made during an interview
5. Formal testing done during the interview

The interview is critical to gathering information about a person's behavior, emotional state, perceptions, and thought processes.

The mental status examination includes assessment of general appearance and behavior, emotional state, perception, thinking, and intellectual functioning.

GENERAL APPEARANCE AND BEHAVIOR

Whenever we assess a resident, it is important to be aware of his or her general appearance, including general bodily characteristics (face, head, neck, eyes, ears, skin, hair, nails, dress, grooming, odors); motor behavior (posture, gait, abnormal movements); problems with autonomic functions (dizziness, dry mouth, palpitations, numbness, tingling, tremors, sweating, flushes), and interaction with the clinician.

EMOTIONAL STATE

During the course of the interview, evaluate the resident's emotional state (i.e., mood and affect). Mood generally refers to how a person describes his own feelings; affect refers to what others observe about the person's mood. To do a mood assessment, ask the resident to rate his mood from 1 to 10, with 1 being low and 10 being high, or ask the resident to describe his mood. (This method will not be useful for persons with advanced dementia.) With the latter approach, you may need to give a list of descriptions (e.g., sad, happy, angry, elated). To assess affect, observe the resident's affective range, intensity, lability, and appropriateness.

Questions to answer include these:

- Are there recent mood or affect changes?
- Does the person have a history of mood or affective disorders?
- Is there acute or chronic confusion (delirium or Alzheimer's disease)?
- Do certain people improve the mood and affect of the resident?

- What does a 24-hour picture of the resident's mood and affect look like? (A behavior monitoring chart is included in Appendix A).
- Is the affect so intense that the resident probably is frequently experiencing catastrophic reactions?
- Are the resident's mood and affect so dulled that he is experiencing excess disability?

It is also important to evaluate whether the subjective and objective assessments of emotional state are congruent. In other words, do you see the person looking depressed although the person denies it?

INTELLECTUAL FUNCTIONING

The purposes of an intellectual assessment are to determine the presence of organic disease—both reversible disease such as delirium and nonreversible disease such as many dementias; monitor changes in the resident's state; and identify the resident's specific strengths and deficits in order to develop an appropriate plan of care.

Evaluation of intellectual functioning includes

- orientation
- old learning
- attention and concentration
- thinking
- memory and recall
- comprehension and judgment
- reading
- writing
- language
- copying

The Folstein Mini Mental State Examination, which is a standard instrument for assessing cognitive function, is in Figure 4.2. When using a mental status questionnaire, remember that you must consider the resident's overall intelligence. Always ask yourself, "Is the wrong response due to cognitive impairment or a low I.Q.?" Also, when testing intellectual functioning, it is important to remember that questioning a resident about his memory or cognitive status may be threatening, making it difficult to gain accurate information.

Ask questions involving judgment and reasoning in the resident's daily life. For example, you might ask, "What would you do if you were walking down the hall and saw another resident fall?" "What would you do if your roommate started choking?" Four aspects of thinking should be assessed:

1. Flow of thoughts—rate, train, or continuity of thought
2. Possession of thoughts—the sense that one's thoughts are one's own and that one is in control of them
3. Content of thoughts (e.g., whether there are delusional disturbances)
4. Form of thoughts (e.g., whether the person's thoughts are logical and with conclusions, coherent, and connected and whether speech is broken)

In the course of a general conversation with the resident, thinking disturbances will often be obvious. A delusion is a false belief or opinion about something. An illusion represents a misinterpretation of an existing object. A hallucination is a visual or auditory perception with no external stimuli. For example, when an individual observes a reflection on the wall of a red curtain as a fire, that is an illusion. If the person says that he sees items on the floor and is trying to pick them up, when nothing is there, that is a hallucination. If someone misperceives an object because of poor vision, that is not an illusion. It is critical to determine whether misperceptions are occurring because of an altered cognitive state or visual deficits. For those residents with less obvious thinking disturbances, asking abstract questions may help elicit the pathology. For example, you might ask

• How are apples and oranges similar?
• How are tables and chairs similar?

Mini Mental State Exam

Instructions: Write down the patient's answer, and also score as (1) correct or (0) incorrect.

1. 1 0	Where are you now? (What place is this? What is the name of this place? What kind of place is it? Ask these questions if necessary to determine if patient knows the name and type of place.)
2. 1 0	What city are we in?
3. 1 0	What county are we in?
4. 1 0	What state are we in?
5. 1 0	What floor are we on?
6. 2 1 0	What is the date today? (e.g., Jan. 21) score 1 point for each
7. 1 0	What year is it?
8. 1 0	What is the day (e.g., Monday)
9. 1 0	What season is it?
10. 3 2 1 0	*Registration*: Ask the patient if you may test his/her memory. Then say "ball," "flag," and "tree" clearly and slowly, about one second for each. After you have said all three, ask patient to repeat them. This first repetition determines the score (0–3), but keep saying the words until patient can repeat all 3, up to 6 trials. If patient cannot learn all 3, recall cannot be tested later. ____ # of trials
11. 5 4 3 2 1 0	*Attention and Calculation*: Ask the patient to begin with 100, and count backwards by 7. Stop after 5 subtractions. Score the total number of correct answers. If the patient cannot or will not perform this task, ask him/her to spell the word "world" backwards. The score is the number of letters in correct order (e.g,. dlrow = 5 dlrow = 3). ____ 93 ____ 86 ____ 79 ____ 72 ____ 65 dlrow
12. 3 2 1 0	*Recall*: Ask the patient to recall the 3 words you previously asked him/her to remember. Score 0–3.

FIGURE 4.2   Mini Mental State Exam.

38

13. 1 0	*Language*: Show patient a wrist watch and ask what it is.
14. 1 0	*Language*: Show patient a pencil and ask what it is.
15. 1 0	*Repetition*: Ask the patient to repeat the sentence: "No ifs, ands, or buts."
16.	*3-Stage Command*: Give subject a piece of blank paper and say, "Take the paper in your right hand, fold it in half, and put it on the floor."
1 0	Takes paper in right hand.
1 0	Folds paper in half.
1 0	Puts paper on floor.
17. 1 0	*Reading*: On a blank piece of paper, print the sentence "Close your eyes," in letters large enough for the patient to see clearly. Ask him/her to do what it says. Score correctly if patient actually closes eyes.
18. 1 0	*Writing*: Give the patient a blank piece of paper and ask him/her to write a sentence. It is to be written spontaneously. It must contain a subject and verb and be sensible. Correct grammar and punctuation are not necessary. Attach to test.
19. 1 0	*Copying*: Give the patient the figure of intersection pentagons, and ask him/her to copy it exactly as it is. All 10 angles must be present and 2 must intersect to score 1 point. Tremor and rotation are ignored.

TOTAL SCORE

_____ 20 or less on Folstein indicates impairment

FIGURE 4.2 (*Continued*)

From Folstein, M., Folstein, S. G., & MuHugh, P. (1975). Mini mental state, a practical method for grading the cognitive state of patients for the clinician. *J Psychiatri Res, 12*, 189–198. Reprinted by permission.

- What does this mean: "People in glass houses shouldn't throw stones?" or "A rolling stone gathers no moss?"

It is important to report findings objectively. A common error is to report interpretations as if they were observations. For example, during an interview a resident may be slow to respond to questions, have slurred speech, and lack direct eye contact. These are objective observations. If the interviewer reports, however, that the resident is "depressed and withdrawn," this might be misleading because the symptoms could be related to physical illness or medication, not depression. Linking symptoms to depression is an interpretation or assessment, not an observation.

None of these assessment approaches, used alone or together, provides a definitive diagnosis. They provide a structured interviewing process that ensures that crucial features of the resident's situation are not overlooked.

The following are examples of documentation of mental status.

Mr. Jordan is a neatly attired, clean-shaven, 82-year-old man. Facial expressions are full, appropriate to the conversation, and coupled with frequent eye contact with the examiner. Varied vocal tones are well modulated, and speech is audible and articulate. Body movements are smooth and coordinated. General affect is one of seriousness accompanied by mild postural tension and intense listening behaviors while symptoms are discussed. Conversation indicates orientation to time, person, place. The client is able to offer logical and reasonable contributions to problem solving and describes past attempts at dealing with his arthritic pain.

Mrs. Thomas is a 65-year-old female who scored 3 correct out of 30 on the Folstein Mini Mental State Exam. She has food stains and food residue on the front of her sweatshirt. Her hair is short, straight, and uncombed in the back. Her facial expression is flat unless engaged in a conversation; then she may occasionally smile or frown appropriately. When she was unable to answer questions on the mental status exam, she became quiet and appeared sad, perhaps indicating some insight into her condition. She paces back and forth in the lounge area and often will follow an individual with whom she has just had a conversation. She appears easily distracted by activity and noises in the environment. She is disoriented to time and place and is unable to state her name but responds with a nod, smile, and "That's it" when her name is spoken. Her speech is sparse and often consists of repeating a word from a preceding question. For example, when asked if she had to go to the bathroom, she replied, with a frown and questioning look, "Go? Go? Go?" She is unable to follow three-step commands or to name objects such as pen and watch.

PSYCHOSOCIAL ASSESSMENT

A psychosocial assessment can provide a better understanding of a resident's psychological and social needs, pertinent history, and recent psychological changes experienced.

Any interventions you choose will have to be based on the resident's strengths and resources. Therefore, a psychosocial assessment should begin by identifying those strengths and resources. Focusing on the positive first prevents seeing the resident purely in terms of a "problem."

In making a psychosocial assessment, it is also important to consider the losses the person has experienced. Loss is a dominant theme in later life, and bereavement overload is common. Bereavement overload occurs when losses come in such rapid succession that before the person has completed the grief work associated with one loss, he experiences another loss. Even the most well-adjusted older person can be overwhelmed by multiple losses and have difficulty coping. Losses may include a spouse, child, friends or relatives, a pet, previously enjoyed activities, vision and/or hearing, ability to drive, a home, a job, mobility, independence, decision making and control, financial security, or health.

These losses place older people at risk for loss of self-worth and self-respect. Often residents may look depressed and, as a result, be started on antidepressants. Antidepressant medications chosen appropriately and given in adequate doses may be very useful. Unfortunately, there are no pills that will increase self-worth or bring back what has been lost. If you have knowledge about what is meaningful to residents and can help them to continue these activities, you will contribute to their well-being. Staff should implement other types of interventions for depresssive symptoms in addition to evaluating the potential effectiveness of medications.

For example, Mrs. Terry loved opera but had a severe hearing loss. However, with headphones and a Walkman-type recorder, she was still able to enjoy her favorite music. Mrs. Zolan, who had dementia, was a housewife and mother. Her restlessness was considerably reduced when she wore an apron that had cleaning rags and a feather duster in the pockets.

Other important aspects to include in a psychosocial assessment are the relevant psychosocial history, current living situation, support systems, financial situation and services currently being used.

A psychological history includes

- sources of pride
- disappointments and regrets
- ways of coping
- sociability
- education
- work
- recent role changes
- social interests
- hobbies
- relationships with family members
- history of psychiatric illness in family
- substance abuse

Assessment of the current living situation includes

- description of current situation (how long in current setting, relationship with roommate, others)
- degree of satisfaction with the situation
- assets and liabilities of the living situation

Support systems to be assessed include

- family
- friends

- fraternal organizations
- religious community
- other organizations

Assessment of the financial situation should include

- financial status
- resident's concerns
- family concerns

Services currently used may include

- social services
- psychiatric services
- medical care
- spiritual support and counseling

SPIRITUAL ASSESSMENT

Occasionally, a resident's behavioral symptoms may stem from unmet spiritual needs. These needs may originate when the person is placed in a nursing home, or nursing home placement may intensify already existing unmet needs. Even under the best of circumstances, moving into a nursing home is a distressing occurrence that adds to one's sense of loss (of independence, belongings, etc.), separation, and isolation. Also, the lack of privacy in a nursing home can be very unsettling, as is the fact that one must accommodate to a group-living situation in which the needs and preferences of others sometimes conflict with one's own.

Assessment of a resident's unmet spiritual needs does not always occur in a formal interview. Rather, this is an interpretive process that unfolds within the context of a trusting relationship. The assessor's nonverbal behavior is very important in establishing and fostering trust. A calm, open, friendly, nonjudgmental, supportive attitude can go a long way toward helping a resident cope with some of the depersonalization inherent in the institutional setting. Questions to guide the overall process of spiritual assessment include these:

- What is this person's religious background?
- What is this person's spirituality?
- What needs are connected with this spirituality?
- How does this person experience/express her spirituality (through music, nature, other people, public worship, private prayer)?

It may be helpful to distinguish between religious preference and spirituality. Religion is a system of beliefs and formal practices that are practiced individually or in community, usually as a focus for finding meaning in life, understanding death, and maintaining hope for the future. Religion is one expression of one's spirituality. Spirituality is an aspect or condition of human beings concerning (1) relationships, involving love and intimacy; (2) meaning and purpose for being; (3) letting go of the crippling past, or forgiveness; (4) openness to the future, and hope (Juan de Fuca Hospitals, 1992). The following may be symptoms of unmet spiritual needs:

- anxiety, fear
- anger, depression
- guilt
- regret, grief
- loneliness, separation, isolation
- need for reconciliation
- lack of positive self-image
- lack of self-identity
- alienation
- questions about the meaning and value of life
- a sense of unfinished business (Kaiser Permanente, 1991).

If a resident has been an active member of a worshipping community, the religious leader of that community may be a good source of information and support.

INTERVENTION

When an assessment is made of a resident's possible unmet spiritual need, several activities are available to help the resident:

- Supportive presence
- Sharing in prayer/Scripture reading (or other inspirational literature
- Offering religious services/worship
- Offering "sacramental rites" (e.g., rituals of healing/reconciliation, anointing)

Any intervention should respect the resident's belief system and promote the resident's autonomy and should be offered from a supportive, not a challenging, stance. Proselytizing is inappropriate.

Ideally, the pastoral task is to encourage and assist the resident in addressing spiritual issues and resolving problems that occur as a result of unmet spiritual needs. This is done by providing occasions or opportunities for the resident to reflect on any aspects of her spirituality and/or religion. Unfortunately, however, some residents may have lost all notion of what their spirituality/religion previously meant to them. In other cases, a resident's behavior may tend to discourage the very caring, compassionate, and supportive presence from staff, family, and friends that is needed or desired. In any event, it is important to remember that while a resident may not express appreciation, she may recognize that sometimes she might be helped most by the regular, reassuring presence of someone whom she trusts.

REFERENCES

Beedle, J. (1991). *The casebook: A workbook for caregivers' peace of mind.* Portland, OR: Lady Bug Press.

Brody, E., Kleban, M., Lawton, M. P., & Silverman, H. (1971). Excess disabilities of mentally impaired aged: Impact of individualized treatment. *Gerontologist, 2,* 124–133.

Juan de Fuca Hospitals, Victoria, BC. (1992). *Pastoral care program: Policies and procedures*. Unpublished manuscript.

Kaiser Permanente Hospice Program, Portland, OR. (1991). *Pastoral care assessment form*. Unpublished manuscript.

Mace, N. (1984). Facets of dementia. *Journal of Gerontological Nursing, 10*(2), 34.

Chapter 5

ASSESSING THE EXTERNAL ENVIRONMENT

Joanne Rader

The environment may be defined as the circumstances, objects, and conditions that surround and affect an individual. In this definition the environment is viewed as external to the individual.

Several authors have developed models that explore the ways in which the environment affects older persons (Kahana, 1974; Kayser-Jones, 1992; Lawton, 1982; Moos & Lemke, 1985) and persons with cognitive impairment (Hall & Buckwalter, 1987).

In one such model, environmental press is the term given to environmental stimuli or characteristics that demand something of the individual. Individual competence is defined as the upper limit of the individual's functional capacity in the areas of biological health, sensation perception, motor behavior, and cognition (Lawton, Windley, & Byerts, 1982). Lawton's model states that as an individual's competencies decrease, the environment, both physical and psychosocial, and the effect of environmental press become more important. That is to say, as a person's competence decreases—as it does with Alzheimer's disease—the person will be more affected by the environment and its demands. In practical terms, this means that the staff and administration must look very closely at the amounts and kinds of stimuli and demands that the nursing home environment creates for residents. The environment thus becomes a helpful intervention that can be manipulated, rather than just a static background that both staff and residents must tolerate. There are a number of excellent books to help with this task. They are included in the "Resource List," Appendix F.

The concept of progressively lowered stress threshold is based on theories of stress and coping and uses resident behavior to determine an appropriate level of environmental stimuli, care, and support to maximize resident safety and comfort (Hall & Buckwalter, 1987). Progressively lowered stress threshold (PLST) can be useful as a framework for assessing possible causes of behavioral symptoms and determining appropriate interventions. Figures 5.1–5.4 illustrate the progressively lowered stress threshold seen in persons with dementia and the effects of different environments.

Persons with dementia have three types of behaviors: baseline, anxious, and dysfunctional. The proportions of these types of behaviors change as the disease progresses. Baseline behaviors include the ability of individuals to communicate in some way and be aware of their surroundings and to function within their limits.

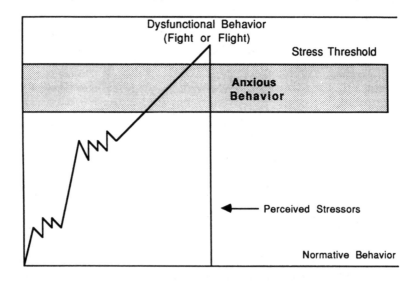

FIGURE 5.1   Stress threshold in normal individuals.

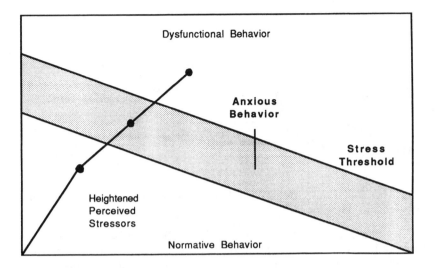

FIGURE 5.2   Progressively lowered stress threshold in adults with progressive degeneration of the cerebral cortex (Alzheimer's disease and related disorders).

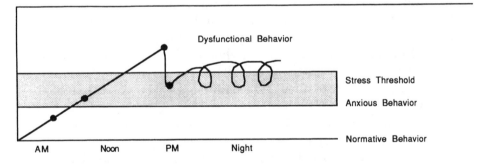

FIGURE 5.3   A typical day for an adult with a dementing illness in an unstructured care program.

These baseline behaviors diminish with the progression of disease and are replaced by anxious and dysfunctional behaviors.

Anxious behaviors are those behaviors that residents demonstrate prior to dysfunctional behaviors. They are clues that the behavior may escalate if no action is taken to decrease stress.

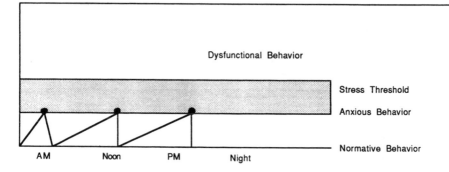

Dysfunctional Behavior

Stress Threshold

Anxious Behavior

Normative Behavior

AM   Noon   PM   Night

FIGURE 5.4 Planned activity levels for the adult with dementing illness.

Figures from Hall, G.R. & Buckwalter, K.C. (1987). Progressively Lowered Stress Threshold: A conceptual Model for Care of Adults with Alzheimer's Disease. *Archives of Psychiatric Nursing*, 1(6), 399–406, Reprinted with permission.

Anxious behaviors will vary from situation to situation and from client to client. Staff reported that one gentleman's very lovely whistling was a sign of increased anxiety, and they knew that if they did not decrease the environmental stress or demands made on him, he would soon be yelling and striking out at staff.

Dysfunctional behaviors occur when individuals experience too many stressors and have no opportunities to relax or decrease stimuli and therefore their stress threshold is exceeded. If it is repeatedly exceeded, the individual cycles between anxious and dysfunctional behavior. The goal is to structure the environment and activities in such a way that staff recognize the anxious behaviors and reduce the stressors, allowing individuals with dementia to stay within their baseline or most nearly normal behavior.

Figure 5.1 illustrates how a normal person may experience stressors that cause him to cross the stress threshold and develop dysfunctional behavior. However, the normal person quickly returns to baseline or normal behavior.

Figure 5.2 shows how, over time, persons with Alzheimer's disease experience a shift so that it takes many fewer events to trigger them into dysfunctional behaviors, thereby lowering the stress threshold. Thus, there is a much greater proportion of dysfunctional behavior to normative behavior than in a normal individual.

Figure 5.3, shows how, with the now lowered stress threshold, the person with dementia often cycles between anxious and dysfunctional behaviors if no one alters the environment to reduce stress. This creates a situation in which the person's normative behaviors are in a sense out of his reach.

However, as shown in Figure 5.4, if staff identify when residents begin anxious behaviors and take action to decrease the environmental stressors, residents are able to return to their baseline behaviors and avoid dysfunctional ones.

The external environment includes organizational, psychosocial, and physical aspects Kayser-Jones (1989). It is critical for the "detective" to explore each of these aspects of the environment when trying to discover clues to the resident's unmet needs that are being expressed as behavioral symptoms (see Figure 5.5).

THE ORGANIZATIONAL ENVIRONMENT

Each corporation, facility, care unit, or shift has its own organizational environment. Elements of the organizational environment include such things as:

- philosophy
- policy and procedures
- staffing patterns
- structure of the day
- staff support and education
- equipment and supplies

Initially, individual caregivers may feel powerless to affect the organizational environment because changes are perceived to occur at a system level, not at the level of the individual worker. However, it is important for caregivers to explore aspects of the organization when looking for causes of resident behavior

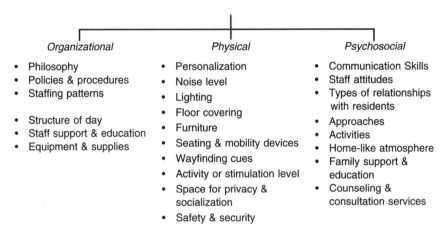

Organizational	Physical	Psychosocial
• Philosophy	• Personalization	• Communication Skills
• Policies & procedures	• Noise level	• Staff attitudes
• Staffing patterns	• Lighting	• Types of relationships with residents
	• Floor covering	
• Structure of day	• Furniture	• Approaches
• Staff support & education	• Seating & mobility devices	• Activities
• Equipment & supplies	• Wayfinding cues	• Home-like atmosphere
	• Activity or stimulation level	• Family support & education
	• Space for privacy & socialization	• Counseling & consultation services
	• Safety & security	

FIGURE 5.5 External environment.

and hoping to engage administration in examining possible system-level problems and changes. In addition, usually each unit and shift create their own organizational environment within the facility. Evaluating the organizational environment for clues about resident behavior and ways to improve the care for residents is productive and exciting. It opens the door to a wide variety of interventions. It challenges administrators to look closely at their policies and philosophy in order to evaluate how these affect behavioral symptoms. It frees staff to be responsive, creative, and caring in ways they may not have previously considered.

Many exemplary organizations have resulted from the initial vision and commitment of one individual who inspired others with the belief that major organizational change was needed and possible. An excellent example of this is change in the use of physical restraints. The recent dramatic changes in practice in this country resulted initially from the work of a small number of committed individuals who, based on their experience and knowledge of other models of care, struggled to make these changes part of the environment of their own organizations and then, on a larger scale, part of the regulatory system (Blakeslee, Goldman, Papougenis, & Torell, 1990; Burger, 1989; Mitchell-Pederson, Edmund, Fingerote, & Powell, 1986; Rader, 1991; Strumpf & Evans, 1991; Williams, 1990).

Philosophy

An organization's philosophy guides practice and priorities. It should reflect a resident-centered, individualized approach. Often facilities lack a philosophy statement or do not translate the statement into action. A good philosophy statement can be used as a standard against which priorities and decisions are judged. For example, Live Oaks Living Center in California has put into practice a philosophy of care that creates a regenerative community in the nursing facility. "Its goal is to synthesize a culture around a value system which fosters the role of the elder among those who live there and which provides tools for expanding the vision of one's potential and capacity to give shape to life" (Barkan, 1981). One way this is operationalized is through daily community meetings in which the residents are engaged in activities such as problem solving, providing mutual support, and creating poetry. A cornerstone of their philosophy is the following definition of an elder:

> An Elder is a person
> who is still growing
> still a learner,
> still with potential and
> whose life continues to have
> within it promise for, and
> connection to the future.
> An Elder is still in pursuit of
> happiness, joy and pleasure,
> and her or his birthright to these
> remains intact. Moreover, an
> Elder is a person who deserves
> respect and honor and whose
> work it is to synthesize wisdom
> from long life experience and
> formulate this into a legacy for
> future generations.

Gråberget Nursing Home in Gothenburg, Sweden, which has an exemplary organizational commitment to individualized care, has the following simple philosophy statement: "All the residents at Gråberget Nursing Home are individuals with their own special needs and desires" (Ulla Turremark, personal communication September 16, 1991).

Questions the "detective" can use in assessing organizational philosophy include these:

- Is there a written philosophy that is resident-centered rather than facility-centered?
- If there is a written philosophy, is it put into practice or is it just words on paper?
- Does the philosophy enhance or inhibit resident autonomy and control?
- Were residents and families involved in developing the philosophy?
- Is the philosophy taught to new employees and included in staff orientation?
- Do training classes for certified nursing assistants teach a resident-centered philosophy?
- Are the certified nursing assistants who have been working many years aware of the facility philosophy and the changes in philosophy mandated by OBRA?
- Have they received education and training related to how the OBRA philosophy affects the way they provide care?

It is also important to identify whether there is an unwritten philosophy contrary to and stronger than the written philosophy.

Policy and Procedures

Policies and procedures may be viewed as a road map for implementing an organization's philosophy. They contain specific information that guides staff in resolving practice issues such as the use of physical restraints and psychoactive medications and in dealing with behaviors thought to be "problematic," such as wandering.

Many of the current policies and procedures in nursing homes were borrowed from the hospital model and have little relevance for current nursing home residents. Mary Lucero (1992) has pointed this out very well. She notes that many facilities have procedures for placing water pitchers at all residents' bedsides. When staff members are asked if many residents actually use this, the answer is no. Staff members often say that residents are more likely to pour the water on their neighbor or use it as a urinal, neither of which is very compatible with maintaining hydration! Persons with dementia are much more likely to remember going to a kitchen sink for a drink than to remember that they have a pitcher at their bedside. It is not "normal" in our own homes to seek a drink at the bedside. It is also not "normal" to go to a drinking fountain in your home. In addition, if the fountain has a push bar, a cognitively impaired resident will generally not know how to use it.

The staff should look to the past and present patterns of the individual to develop a plan. It may be quite possible to do away with the water pitcher policies and procedures and address hydration needs individually. Mr. Stevens, for example, was occasionally using his water pitcher as a urinal. The staff also observed that he would frequently pick up glasses and cups from other residents' trays and drink from them. They determined that the needs underlying his behaviors were (1) assistance with toileting and (2) quenching his thirst. Because they had observed that on one occasion he tried to drink from a urinal, they decided against placing a urinal at the bedside. Instead, they provided frequent prompting to use the toilet and offered him cranberry juice (his favorite drink) during the morning and afternoon social activity, which he liked to attend. They removed the water pitcher from the bedside and brought to the attention of the administration that there was a need to reexamine the routine procedure of placing water at the bedside.

Another example of inappropriate policies pointed out by Lucero (1992) involves the use of call lights. Few residents with cognitive impairment know how to use the call light system. Sometimes call lights may even be hazardous, for example, if residents get the cords around their necks or extremities. Lucero describes an often-repeated scene in which the state surveyors are coming up the walk and the staff is frantically pinning call lights to the chests of comatose residents. They do so because in the past surveyors asked the staff why the individuals did not have a call light within reach. When they were told that a person was unable to use the system, they said to give it to them anyway. Under the new OBRA philosophy, this is much less likely to happen. The policy of ensuring that all residents have call lights within reach is changed now. Instead, all residents should have an identified way in which they are able to let staff members know of their needs and have those needs met. For example, for a person who is comatose, the individualized plan may be that all staff members will observe the person as they walk by the room, particularly observing to see whether the person is correctly positioned and showing no signs of distress in breathing patterns and expression in the eyes, and the aide assigned to the person will check on her every 30 minutes. For some residents, calling out "Nurse!" is the way they alert staff.

The policy of scheduling baths only on specific days and shifts also needs to be reevaluated. Mrs. Mantor, who had dementia, would awake on some mornings in a cooperative, pleasant mood. The nursing assistant knew that on these days she would be agreeable to showering. If the shower was attempted on an uncooperative day, she became quite verbally and physically aggressive. The staff altered their care plan so the shower would occur only on the mornings when the nursing assistant determined that Mrs. Mantor was cooperative. The shower experience was altered to fit the individual's needs and ability to cope, not determined by an assigned day of the week.

It behooves facilities to critically examine all current polices and procedures for their relevance and efficiency. A great deal of time, energy, and money are wasted in routines that have no relevance for the current nursing home population.

Staffing Patterns

The staffing patterns most frequently used in long-term care settings are based on an acute care hospital model and frequently do not meet the needs of residents. It is almost as if we expected all residents to be going for surgery in the morning: we staff heavily on the day shift and have fewer people on evening and night shifts.

Yet the great majority of nursing home residents have some form of dementia, and many become more fatigued, confused, restless, and distressed in the evening hours, when many facilities have significantly lighter staffing and fewer activities. Another frequently used approach to care is to assign staff to specific tasks rather than to residents. There are bath aides, restorative aides, feeding aides, and so on. This provides little security or support for residents with memory loss.

One concept that holds great promise for improving the quality of life for nursing home residents and staff alike is that of permanent assignments. Permanent assignments mean that staff on each shift work with the same residents over a long period of time. This is in contrast to the common practice of rotating staff from resident group to resident group and sometimes even from unit to unit. In one permanent assignment model (Tedros, 1992), permanent consistent staff included certified nursing assistants (CNAs), nurses and housekeeping, and dietary staff. Facilities have reported less resident distress and dramatic improvements in residents' overall sense of security and comfort when permanent assignments for CNAs were established (Beryl Goldman, personal communication, August 18, 1992; Lucero, 1992; Mace, 1993). A permanent staffing structure supports the development of relationships between the staff, resident, and family. Facilities that use permanent staff assignments report that residents, families, and staff prefer this.

There are pros and cons to this approach, however. Initially, some facilities have reported staff resistance to making the change. For example, one facility in Canada reported that several CNAs felt they couldn't "stand" to take care of the same group for more than 3 days. This raises the question of what it must feel like for residents to be cared for by someone with this attitude. Perhaps staff members feel that way because they are forced to function in an organizational environment poorly designed to meet the client's needs. This same group of CNAs, when encouraged to make a first step toward more stable assignments and stop rotating from unit to unit, found that they were very pleased with the change (Monahan, personal communication, September 23, 1993).

To overcome this possible initial resistance, it is helpful to negotiate a plan for a limited trial with periodic evaluations so that staff members feel that the change is a process in which their input is critical. However, at times it is important for administration to take a firm stand. One director of nursing reported that generally the staff in her facility was pleased with the change to permanent assignments. However, a nurse on the evening shift on one unit was not supportive of the change, and the CNAs also did not like it. This was the same unit that had had most difficulty in eliminating the use of restraints. The director of nursing, basing her decision on the positive response to permanent assignments from the rest of the staff and her knowledge of this individual nurse's general reluctance to change, responded to the staff's resistance by telling the nurse and CNAs that until they could clearly state how the old way of rotating assignments was better for the resident, she was unwilling to listen. As with eliminating the use of physical restraints, often staff reluctance to change is the biggest impediment to improving practice.

Staff members who have been on permanent assignments report the following positive results: There is a more predictable flow to the daily schedule; they get to know the residents better; resident anxiety and restlessness decrease; staff members recognize when the residents begin to get agitated and know what specific things will calm them; families know whom to contact if they want something done; personal items such as clothing, glasses, and teeth are less often lost; and there is more time to do special things for residents.

Problems that have been encountered with permanent assignment include a sense of territory and ownership on the part of the staff, painful grieving upon the death of residents one has cared for, CNAs who make decisions for residents, and a feeling of burnout with difficult residents. Most of these problems, however, can be dealt with by anticipating them and developing a plan for managing them.

Questions you may wish to ask about staffing patterns include these:

- Is the facility using standard staffing patterns, or is the staff exploring alternative ways of staffing to meet the unique needs of the residents and unit?

- Are staff members assigned specific tasks (such as bathing or restorative care), or are they assigned to specific residents?
- Do staff members view their jobs as completing a series of tasks or as enhancing the quality of a resident's day?

Structure of the Day

In general, residents tend to do better and feel more secure if there is some structure and predictability to their daily lives. This is particularly true of persons with dementia. Structure refers to the general flow of the daily schedule. When residents lack a sense of predictability in the flow of their days, this can lead to fear, irritation, and distress. Consequently, it is critical to look at the flow of each resident's day to see if a lack of appropriate programs and activities could be the unmet need that is being expressed behaviorally. It is important, however, to make a distinction between providing a predictable flow to the day and being inflexible. Inflexibility and rigidity in regard to the times when tasks must be done can create stress for both resident and staff and result in discomfort, anxiety, and fear, which in turn produce behavioral reactions distressing to the individual, other residents, and staff.

Mr. Jones, a person with Alzheimer's disease, illustrates this point. Mr. Jones had had a lifelong habit of awakening at 9 a.m. Sometimes he was not ready to get up at 9. Staff found that if they insisted he get up, Mr. Jones became agitated and lashed out at them. If they went away and assisted someone else for 15 minutes to a half hour, he awakened calmly, and the morning routine was accomplished smoothly.

If residents choose to sleep later and miss breakfast, there should be a simple, easy-to-fix substitute such as cold cereal or microwaved oatmeal to offer them upon arising. Staff members sometimes feel that if they allow a resident to miss breakfast or refuse it, they are at risk for criticism by surveyors for violating the regulation that meals must be offered no more than 14 hours apart. However, if it is the resident's wish and he shows no untoward weight loss that needs further assessment, this approach reflects the resident's right to choose. The regulation refers to the responsibility of the facility to offer meals routinely, not that the facility is responsible for having all residents eat in that time frame.

Questions to ask about the structure of the day include these:

- Are residents encouraged to sleep, eat, and get up in their familiar daily patterns, or is there pressure to conform to schedules established by the staff or the institution?
- Is there a predictable, comfortable rhythm and flow to the day for residents?
- Is there flexibility in the structure of the day to accommodate resident changes and preferences?
- Are periods of structured activities alternated with periods of quiet and rest?

Staff Support and Education

A vital part of the organizational environment is the way in which the system supports the staff. An organization cannot expect its staff to treat residents with any more care and respect than the staff receives from administrators. Regulators, including surveyors, complaint investigators, and ombudsmen, also have opportunities to model respect and support when interacting with both staff and residents. Questions to ask to determine if there is appropriate staff support include these:

- Do staff members have access to resources that enhance their caregiving skills, such as books, consultants, and educational programs?
- Are staff members encouraged to attend workshops by having paid in-service days and workshop fees paid by the facility?
- Does the supervisory staff have expertise in staff management?
- What provisions are made to provide support, debriefing, and problem solving for staff members who have been involved in an aggressive/combative situation with a resident?

- Are in-services routinely offered that explore ways to defuse and prevent aggression and handle other difficult situations?
- Are geriatric mental health consultants available to the staff for problem solving and education?
- Are the Minimum Data Set (MDS) Manual and Resident Assessment Protocols (RAPS) and triggers available for use in each unit?
- Do surveyors, ombudsmen, and administrators seek staff input, perceptions, and opinions, along with those of residents and families?
- Is there an employee assistance program available for staff members experiencing an emotional or financial crisis?
- Are the numbers and expertise of the staff generally sufficient?

Equipment and Supplies

One way in which the administration can support staff members is by assuring that they have up-to-date and adequate equipment and supplies. For example, one fairly common problem is insufficient linen. The cause of this is often complex. Sometimes staff members from one shift "hide and hoard" linen to assure adequate amounts on their shift. In addition, there may be inadequate amounts of linen or problems getting it returned in a timely manner from the laundry. It is important to address supply issues.

With the decrease in the use of physical restraints comes a need for different types of equipment and supplies to create alternatives to restraints (see chapter 10). The cost of these alternatives overall is low (Restraint Minimization Project, 1993), but some facilities have found administrators reluctant to see that a new need exists. Administrators need to consider these questions:

- Are adequate supplies routinely available to the staff?
- Are administrators and staff aware of the latest innovations in care equipment?
- Is there a plan for systematically upgrading equipment?
- Is the current equipment in good working order?

THE PHYSICAL ENVIRONMENT

The relationship of the physical environment of the nursing home to residents' behavioral symptoms is an exciting area to explore. Modifying the physical environment to meet individuals' needs can positively influence behaviors.

The physical environment should support and enhance the normal experiences of daily living through such means as contact with food preparation, its sounds and scents; a homelike setting for TV watching or people watching; groups of small tables and chairs for socializing; and variety in design, color, and texture.

Many nursing homes have done much to create a more comforting and homelike environment. Some have also developed special care units to meet the needs of persons with dementia. Aspects of the physical environment to assess include these:

- Personalization
- Noise level
- Lighting
- Floor covering
- Furniture
- Seating and mobility devices
- Way-finding cues
- Activity or stimulation level
- Space for privacy and socialization
- Safety and security

Personalization

Opportunities to personalize one's immediate surroundings contribute to a sense of well-being. Personal objects are symbols of past adventures, roles, and connections. A personalized environment makes a statement about who a person is, allows a person to stake out a territory, helps a person maintain his identity, and provides orienting cues for a person with confusion (Calkins, 1988).

Questions to ask about personalization include these:

- Is the environment personalized appropriately for the resident?
- Are personal items safe, or are they at risk of becoming lost or stolen?
- Can residents bring in their own beds, chairs, pictures, and chest of drawers?
- Do they have the freedom to put pictures on the walls and personalize bedspreads and window coverings?

Noise Level

Staff and frequent visitors to nursing facilities may become desensitized to the noise level and the role that noise plays in creating difficult behaviors. Many residents, because of cognitive or physical impairment, lack the ability to screen out or escape from environmental noise. Others are particularly sensitive to constant noise or the jarring noise from intercoms. Questions to ask that can assist staff in understanding noise as a source of difficulty include these:

- What is the usual noise level on the nursing unit, during activities, during change of shift, and at night?
- Have any attempts been made to decrease the noise level?
- Does the resident respond negatively to high noise levels?
- How is the intercom system used? Have ways to eliminate or decrease its use been explored?
- Are music and tapes of the resident's choice used routinely and therapeutically to create a relaxed, quiet environment?
- Are staff members' shoes noisy, especially during quiet times and at night?
- Are carts, wheelchairs, and other equipment in need of maintenance to decrease noisiness?
- Is a TV contributing only noise and confusion to the environment?
- Do open windows bring in pleasant or unpleasant outdoor noises?

Mr. Jaspar illustrates the effects of noise. He was a violinist, and his greatest pleasure was listening to tapes of the orchestra in which he had played. He gave up listening to the tapes because the intercom spoiled the concerts. Then he grew depressed. The facility learned from this and began using an individual beeper system instead of the intercom. Mr. Jasper's spirits improved, and he began listening to tapes again. Other residents were calmer too.

Lighting

Lighting affects comfort, safety, and the ability to function. Changes in the aged eye require special consideration. The average nursing home resident is over the age of 80, and people at this age require three times more light than a 20-year-old does to perform the same tasks (Christenson, 1990a). In addition, the ability to tolerate glare from windows and reflections from any shiny surface, such as floors, decreases as we age.

Areas to explore related to lighting include these:

- Is the lighting in halls adequate?
- Is there sufficient light for reading?
- Are the fluorescent lights working properly, not flickering?
- Are desk lamps and table lamps available to provide extra lighting, soften the effect of fluorescent bulbs, and create a more homelike appearance and feeling?
- Do the residents have adequate lighting in their rooms to allow them to engage in favorite activities such as reading and crafts?
- Is furniture placed so that natural light can be used as much as possible?
- Do windows and window coverings let light in but minimize glare?

Floor Coverings

There are two major types of floor coverings, vinyl and carpet. Vinyl may be so shiny that it creates glare and contributes to falls.

Some facilities have moved away from vinyl to carpeting. In the past, carpeting was considered problematic because of incontinence, spills, and odor. However, the new carpets have improved backing and are easier to clean. Carpeting helps with noise abatement, it reduces glare and may decrease the risk of injury related to falls, and it contributes to a more homelike atmosphere. Carpets should be low-looped, tightly woven, and of dense pile. The type of floor covering can affect ambulation for some residents because of their assistive devices, gait, or shoes; these need to be taken into account when making decisions.

Questions to ask related to floor coverings include these:

- Does the resident have the appropriate shoes and walker for his gait and the floor covering?
- Is the floor so shiny that the glare may be hard on residents' eyes or create reflections that confuse them?

A number of facilities have moved away from maintaining a high shine on vinyl flooring. One facility developed a "decline of the shine" committee to explore low-gloss finishes and buffing methods. This resulted in reducing the glare from the vinyl floors. Because the housekeeping staff and often the public equate high shine with cleanliness, it is critical to reeducate people to understand that a low-gloss floor better meets the needs of the residents who live there and it is just as clean.

Furniture

The appropriate type, size, and placement of furniture can greatly improve resident function. The height of the bed is especially significant. Many nursing home beds are too high to permit the resident's feet to touch the floor while seated at the edge, creating an unsafe environment and restricting the person's ability to achieve her greatest functional independence.

The type and size of chairs (lounge and side chairs and recliners) and sofas used in a facility can inhibit or enhance function and comfort. Specific information is available to guide staff in choosing appropriate seating (see Christenson, 1990b). Seating should be individualized, using the correct chair size and cushions and supports. Generally, however, facilities choose chairs all of one size, and these do not suit the needs of many residents. Moreover, furniture on wheels, often used by residents for support, can be dangerous.

Questions to ask about furniture include these:

- Is the furniture the best size and arrangement for residents' individual needs?
- Do residents' feet firmly touch the ground when seated at the bedside?
- Are there unstable objects or furniture with wheels in the environment that need to be removed or made safer for support?
- Are a variety of different sizes of chairs available?
- Does the arrangement of furniture in common areas promote socialization?
- Are toilets and commodes the right height?
- Are drawers easily opened, without falling out of the dresser or bedside stand?

Seating and Mobility Devices

With our increasing focus on resident well-being and decreased use of physical restraints, the importance of seating and mobility has become clearer. Facilities are charged with assisting residents to achieve their highest practicable level of function. Yet we restrict mobility and comfort not only by what we place on an individual as a restraint but also by what we do not provide for them.

For example, the standard wheelchair used for nursing home residents is the collapsible, sling-back, sling-seat chair. This chair was designed originally for transportation only; it was not meant to be used as the primary seating for residents. This type of chair generally does not enhance comfort or function. Behavioral symptoms labeled as agitation and restlessness may well be caused by an ill-fitting or uncomfortable chair, so it is important for "detectives" to examine seating as a possible external cause of distress and difficult behavior.

One discipline alone cannot possibly have all the information needed to select the most useful and practical, least costly devices for a frail individual; therefore, an interdisciplinary team approach should be used to assess seating and mobility needs. As a rule of thumb, if any one type of device is used extensively, you need to question whether you are actually individualizing care, because the population's needs are very diverse (see chapter 12).

General questions to ask about seating and mobility include these:

- Do the wheelchairs have sling or firm seats and backs?
- Has an interdisciplinary team assessed seating and mobility needs?
- Do the residents look and feel comfortable in their chairs?
- Do residents complain?
- Do residents appear restless?
- Are a variety of sizes and shapes of chairs available, as well as methods to custom fit as needed?
- Are a variety of walkers available and being used?
- Are the bed heights adjustable? If not, are there other methods to lower the bed if necessary (mattress on floor, low bed frame)?
- Are the shoes that residents wear appropriate and safe?
- Does each resident have an easy chair of his own selection in his room?

Chapter 12 discusses the importance of comfortable seating.

Way-Finding Cues—Landmarks and Signs

There are a variety of ways in which the environment can provide guidance to residents and others in finding their way around the facility. Landmarks and signs increase the sense of security and can

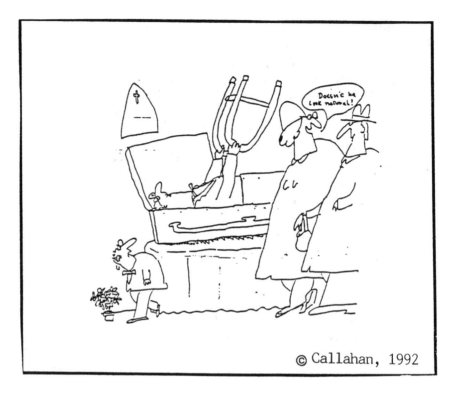

© Callahan, 1992

minimize anxiety in residents. Landmarks include objects such as pictures, wall hangings, and furnishings that aid in navigating the facility.

Signs should be easy to read. Dark words on a light background with letters at least 2–3 inches high are easiest for older persons to distinguish (Calkins, 1988).

The location of signs should take into account the smaller, stooped stature, reduced vision, and decreased upward gaze of older persons and those residents who navigate by wheelchair. Signs should be placed no higher than $4^{1}/_{2}$ feet above the floor and as low as 2 inches above the handrail (Christenson, 1990a). Questions to ask about way-finding cues include these:

- Is the resident's room personalized enough to provide orientation cues?

- Are there cues in the environment that distinguish one unit from another?
- Do signs in the facility direct you to where you want to go?
- Are letters on signs large enough and spaced well enough so that older persons can easily read them?
- Are signs located at the right height?
- Does the sign indicating a resident's room meet her particular needs? (These may change over time.)

Activity or Stimulation Level

Activity level refers to the general level and quality of stimulation in the environment. Some areas have a peaceful, calm feeling; others are anxious and chaotic.

Time of day contributes greatly to activity level. Generally, activity level is higher at change of shift. If staff members are anxious, angry, or upset during this time (perhaps someone did not show up for work), the overall activity level and feel of the unit can create restlessness and agitation among the residents.

If residents are anxious or restless, it is important to observe the general activity level and mood of the unit and consider how these might affect behavior. Several simple interventions can quickly create a calmer level, for example, playing quiet music, turning off the TV (if no resident is watching it), or having staff lower their voices. Often staff habits of yelling back and forth and speaking loudly and abruptly to residents are prime contributors to confusion and discomfort. Consider these:

- Is there a relationship between unit activity level and the residents' behavior?
- What can be done to create a less chaotic, calmer environment?

Space for Privacy and Socialization

The opportunity to make decisions about privacy and social contact is important in every person's life. It can be especially important for institutionalized persons who have lost control of so many other aspects of their lives. The opportunity for residents to have some control or perceived control over social interaction is important. (Calkins, 1988)

Mr. Smith illustrates this point. He came back from a day's outing with his good friends. They walked him to his room to chat because they would not be seeing him for a while. The three of them walked into his room, which he shared with two other residents. A CNA was changing the pants of one of his roommates in his space. The soothing effect of the day was quickly lost as the resident being changed struggled with modesty. The guests were horrified, and Mr. Smith cried in sadness and anger.

Many nursing home residents engage in null behavior, which is the lack of any observable behavior or activity. Of course, everyone enjoys periods of "doing nothing" and "staring," but when this behavior is continuous, it is cause for investigation. Null behavior is most likely to occur when residents do not have the opportunity to choose between privacy and socialization. Providing opportunities for both privacy and social interaction decreases the incidence of null behavior. Interestingly, when opportunities for privacy are provided, social interaction increases (Calkins, 1988). This may be because if there are no opportunities for privacy in the physical environment, the resident establishes privacy by reducing contact with others. Therefore, the staff needs to develop skill in creating opportunities for both privacy and socialization and support residents' choices related to these. One way to do this is to create "Do Not Disturb" signs and make them available for residents and families to place on the door when they wish to be alone or undisturbed. This, of course, would need to be coordinated with any roomates.

Areas to explore include these:

- Are there spaces and opportunities for residents to have privacy?
- Does the arrangement of furniture promote interaction?
- Can the schedule of activities be adjusted to create private times for residents who are in double or multiple-roommate rooms?

- Is there a space in the facility that can be used for privacy needs?
- Do the residents display null behavior, and could that be related to lack of privacy and socialization?

Safety and Security

Safety and security refer to the degree to which the environment is designed to prevent accidents while not inhibiting ease of locomotion (Calkins, 1988). For persons with cognitive impairment, it may be necessary to establish areas with different degrees of access (Calkins, 1988):

- No access to areas of the environment that contain hazards (medicine rooms, maintenance closets)
- Limited access to areas that contain potential hazards but can be made safe with supervision
- Unlimited access to other areas so that residents are able to move, touch, and roam freely

Questions to ask about safety and security include these:

- Are areas of no access secure?
- Have resident areas been assessed for safety?
- Are there areas where residents can safely roam, touch, and explore?
- Does the facility have a safety committee to problem-solve environmental safety issues and to put safety and reasonable risk taking in an appropriate perspective?

THE PSYCHOSOCIAL ENVIRONMENT

When asked, residents indicate that what matters most to them is that they are treated with dignity, respect, kindness, and consideration. Therefore, the most important aspect of creating a positive environment in the nursing home is creating a positive psychosocial environment. The psychosocial environment reflects staff communication skills, staff attitudes, staff willingness to nurture healthy relationships, staff approaches to behavior, the structure of activities, the nursing home atmosphere, family support and education, and counseling and consultation services.

COMMUNICATION SKILLS

The ability to identify and use skillful communication is key to understanding behavioral symptoms. The way that the staff communicates to residents, both verbally and nonverbally, is crucial. Residents with dementia often have decreased verbal abilities and difficulty understanding the meaning of what is said to them. In a sense, they "speak" and understand a different language. Therefore, the task for staff is to learn the language of dementia.

For some demented residents, behavior is the primary means of communicating; this is particularly likely in the later stages of dementing illness. As their verbal abilities deteriorate, persons with dementia become more sensitive to the nonverbal behavior of others. For example, the meaning of "relax" will not be understood if it is said in a tense voice. A resident may become tearful or resist care if he senses that the staff member is angry or hurried. Therefore, another task of staff is to analyze how their communication may affect a resident's behavior. Chapter 13 discusses communication skills in more detail. Important information to gather about communication includes the following:

- What are the residents' communication difficulties if any?
- Does the way the staff and others communicate to residents enhance or inhibit their function?
- How did the family communicate with the resident prior to admission?
- What can family members teach staff members about communicating with the resident?
- How skillful is the staff in communicating verbally?
- How skillful is the staff in communicating nonverbally?

- Are verbal and nonverbal messages congruent?
- Does the resident have specific ways of communicating that only a few staff members understand?

Staff Attitudes

Staff attitudes are a part of communication, but they are so important that they warrant a separate evaluation. Staff attitudes reflect both the individual's approach and the organizational environment. Staff attitudes include how staff members view their jobs, whether or not the staff values residents and relationships with residents, and how the staff perceives and responds to difficult resident behaviors.

Things to consider about staff attitudes include these:

- Do staff members view difficult behavior as a problem or as reflecting an unmet need?
- Does the resident's behavior vary with different staff members who have different attitudes?
- Are staff members willing to look at ways of changing their behaviors and approaches?
- Do staff members seem to "blame" the resident for difficult behavior, or do they look for causes of problems outside the resident?
- Does the staff talk about residents in their presence?
- Do staff members tease residents or make fun of behavioral symptoms?

Nurturing Healthy Relationships

A healthy relationship is one in which both parties' autonomy and individuality are respected and supported. Those involved are considered to be partners. One factor that seems to inhibit our ability to individualize care is the "we-they" approach to relationships with residents: "we" are boss, and "they" are lucky that we are here to help. Paul Managan (1993) describes this phenomenon in his talk titled "Do Old People Come from Outer Space?" Managan observes that caregivers frequently act as if aged people are "beamed down" from outer space, prewrinkled. This, of course, means that the phenomenon of aging will not occur in "normal" people like nurses, doctors, and family members. It has been reported that in European countries (such as England and Scotland) relationships with residents are more normal; the elders are treated as neighbors, friends, or the mothers and fathers of friends and less like "patients," even when they suffer from dementia (VanSon, personal communication, June 24, 1991).

A much more effective and healthy relationship is created when caregivers recognize the equality of residents and empower them by viewing residents' care needs and wishes as central to their job. However, doing too much for residents can be harmful if they are capable of doing things for themselves. Therefore, considerable skill is needed to nurture healthy relationships. Things to consider in assessing staff nurturing of healthy relationships include these:

- Is the staff aware of ways to support residents' autonomy?
- Is sitting and talking to residents viewed as part of the job or as a way to avoid work?

Staff Approaches

Staff approaches refer to how staff members choose to systematically handle a particular behavioral symptom or situation or try to prevent the behavior or situation from occurring. The staff needs to be aware that very little of the physically aggressive behaviors of persons with dementia is spontaneous or part of their normal behavior. Most physically aggressive behaviors occur in response to intrusion into the individual's personal space by staff or other residents and is a defensive response to a perceived threat rather than an expression of anger (Bridges-Parlet, Knopman, & Thompson, 1994). The staff's approach reflects the interplay of various parts of the organizational, physical, and psychosocial environment. It includes elements of communication, attitudes, environment, structure of the day, and activities. Questions to ask about staff approaches include these:

- Do staff members clearly identify specific behavioral symptoms?
- Do staff members explore internal and external factors in determining underlying causes of behavior?
- If the cause cannot be eliminated, what alternative "tools" or approaches decrease the behavior?
- Is there a systematic plan for addressing specific situations considered problematic by the staff?
- Were the resident and/or family involved in developing the plan?

Activities

It is important to think of activities in a broad sense, not just as tasks or functions done by the activity department. Activities are also the events that fill one's day, such as eating, dressing, straightening up the environment, gazing out the window, and being outdoors.

Information about a resident's previous activity patterns and interests can provide valuable clues to whether current activities are meeting the resident's needs. Residents who are not cognitively impaired are generally able to say clearly whether or not current programs and activities are meeting their needs, so they should be asked. Frequently, these individuals may have physical limitations that led to their nursing home placement. It may be that the things they like to do are no longer possible for them or may require some adaptation.

With the cognitively impaired, the staff sometimes needs to "listen" to their behavior to determine whether activities are appropriate and meeting their needs. For example, Mr. Simpson, who had dementia, was restless and had a history of wandering at home and at the nursing home. He was quite content during the day, when he was occupied with activities and just observing and interacting with others in the usual unit activities. However, during the evening his wandering increased, and he once climbed over the fence of the enclosed courtyard. Investigation revealed that this occurred after dinner when the CNAs were in others' rooms preparing them for bed and the nurse was on her supper break. It appeared that when he was all alone in the lounge, his restlessness and insecurity increased and he felt a need to leave to seek security. His history revealed that he had worked in the post office sorting mail for many years. He also had been observed in the nursing home taking papers off the desk. The staff developed a plan that included collecting junk mail and presenting it to him in a box at a table during the evening hours. In addition, they assigned a different nursing assistant to check his whereabouts every 15 minutes and compliment him on the good job he was doing. This resolved his evening wandering and jaunts over the fence. He was able to do an activity that was familiar, and this increased his self-esteem.

Areas to explore in relation to activities include these:

- What were the events that filled each resident's day prior to nursing home placement?
- Is the resident encouraged to continue usual home maintenance activities (dusting, organizing, bedmaking, decorating)?
- Are activities adapted to the resident's current level of function?
- What remaining strengths of the resident could activities build on?

Several models provide guidance about possible ways to structure activities for residents with dementia (Lucero, 1992; Zgola, 1987). These models can be used to assess whether the activities currently in place in your facility are meeting resident needs.

The Nursing Home Atmosphere

Creating a homelike environment involves much more than personalizing the environment. Carboni (1990) sees the experience of home and homelessness as a continuum. Home is where a strong, intimate, fluid relationship exists between the individual and the environment, and homelessness is where the relationship between the individual and the environment is tenuous and severely damaged. Carboni argues that many nursing home residents feel homeless because the true attributes of a home are often lost in the nursing home. Those attributes include the experience of departing and returning, lived space, identity, connectedness, privacy, power/autonomy, and safety/predictability.

Carboni (1990) takes the concept of homelike atmosphere far beyond pictures on the wall and nicely painted and papered walls. She states that the pain of feeling homeless following nursing home placement may be so profound that nursing home residents often cope with it by "pretending" they have adjusted to institutionalization. In addition, family and staff may use denial that the resident's pain exists as a way to avoid their own discomfort.

A study done in Sweden (Zingmark, Norberg, & Sandman, 1993) describes the experience of at-homeness and homesickness in persons with Alzheimer's disease and emphasizes the importance of a personalized physical environment, as well as staff that is skillful in creating for residents a sense of being "at home" and emotionally

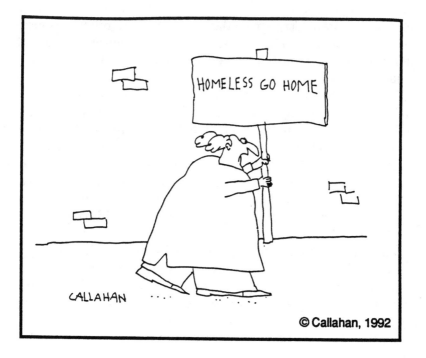

© Callahan, 1992

related to staff members—to the point of wanting to sit close to caregivers and sometimes even on the caregiver's lap.

Asking the resident, "What makes a good day for you?" and "What makes a bad day for the you?" (Williams, personal communication, September 15, 1992) can be very helpful. Additional questions to ask about the homelike quality of the environment include these:

- Does the resident feel that he is homeless? If so, what contributes to this feeling?
- What can be done to increase the attributes of "home" for residents?
- Are staff members encouraged to show affection toward residents?

Family Support and Education

Nursing home placement has been viewed as a time when care and decisions are transferred from the resident and family to the facility and staff. Therefore, families are often uncertain about their role after admission. In addition, they struggle with the guilt and loss frequently associated with the move.

As we move toward a model of long-term care in which the nursing home is viewed more as a part of the community, the role and focus of the family must change. Both the resident and family must be included in decision-making and care activities, and interdependence must be encouraged among all members of the community (Kari & Michels, 1991). How the family view their roles and how they are educated and supported are determined, in large part, by the organizational environment and philosophy of the facility.

Facilities may have formal or informal support systems for families, or both. Many facilities have regular meetings or family forums. Most have some type of informal system to help families who visit routinely get to know each other and provide mutual support.

Important questions to ask include these:

- Are educational opportunities provided for families, such as regular meetings?
- Have residents and families been helped to understand that their input is vital to good care and resident well-being?
- Have the resident and/or family been asked about their wishes regarding involvement in care activities and decision making?
- Have those wishes been honored?
- Have families been encouraged to remain involved in caregiving?
- What type of support system exists for families?
- What formal support is available?
- How effective is the level or type of support provided?
- What is done to facilitate informal and formal networks?
- Is there a family council that meets routinely?

Counseling and Consultation Services

Many nursing home residents suffer from multiple losses and diminished coping resources, and they lack a significant other with whom to talk. Many experience situational depression that might respond to counseling, or major depressive episodes that might respond to medications and counseling.

In addition, a very high percentage of nursing home residents have some form of dementia, and many of these exhibit behavioral symptoms, such as aggression toward staff and others. There is a tremendous need for mental health counseling and consultation in nursing homes. However, the staff often does not have access to good consultation.

Ideally, every facility should have access to a skilled mental health clinician who is interested, experienced, and knowledgeable about geriatric mental health issues. Because psychiatric help or counseling is often threatening to residents, the clinician may need to alter her approach accordingly.

The consultant also needs to be aware of the unique nature of the nursing home structure when making suggestions about interventions and approaches so that these are practical and realistic (Ingersoll-Dayton & Rader, 1993).

Questions to ask about consultation include these:

- Does the facility have an identified mental health consultant?
- Are mental health or psychiatric consultations pursued when appropriate?
- Would one be useful?
- Would the resident or family benefit from a therapeutic group?
- Is counseling available through insurance, the church, or mental health clinics?
- Are there other residents or families who have had similar difficulties who could serve as a support to the resident or family?

REFERENCES

Barkan, B. (1981, Sept–Oct.). The Live Oak Regenerative Community: Reconnecting culture with the long term care environment. *Aging*, pp. 2–7.

Blakeslee, J., Goldman, B., Papougenis, D., & Torell, C. (1990). Debunking the myths. *Geriatric Nursing, 11*(6), 290.

Bridges-Parlet, S., Knopman, D., & Thompson, T. (1994). A descriptive study of physically aggressive behavior in dementia by direct observation. *Journal of American Geriatric Society, 42*, 192–197.

Burger, S. (1989). Inappropriate use of chemical and physical restraints: An ombudsman's resource paper for effective advocacy. Washington, DC: American Association of Retired Persons (AARP) Press.

Calkins, M. (1988). *Design for dementia: Planning environments for the elderly and the confused.* Owings Mills, MD: National Health Publishing.

Carboni, J. (1990). Homelessness among the institutionalized elderly. *Journal of Gerontological Nursing, 16*, 32–37.

Christenson, M. (1990a). Guidelines for selecting landmarks and signage. In E. Taira (Ed.), *Aging in the designed environment* (pp 113–123). New York: Haworth Press.

Christenson, M. (1990b). Chair design and selection for older adults. In E. Taira (Ed.), *Aging in the designed environment* (pp 67–85). New York: Haworth Press.

Hall, G. R., & Buckwalter, K. C. (1987). Progressively lowered stress threshold: A conceptual model for care of adults with Alzheimer's disease. *Archives of Psychiatric Nursing, 1*, 399–406.

Ingersoll Dayton, B., & Rader, J. (1993). Searching for solutions: Mental health consultation in nursing homes. *Clinical Gerontologist, 13*(1), 33–49.

Kahana, E. (1974). Matching environments to needs of the aged: A conceptual scheme. In J. F. Gubrium (Ed.), *Late life: Communities and environmental policy*. Springfield, IL: Charles C. Thomas.

Kari, N., & Michels, P. (1991). The Lazarus project: The politics of empowerment. *American Journal of Occupational Therapy, 45*, 719–725.

Kayser-Jones, J. (1989). The environment and quality of life in long-term care institutions. *Nursing and Health Care, 10*(3), 125–130.

Kayser-Jones, J. (1992). Cultural environment and restraints: A conceptual model for research and practice. *Journal of Gerontological Nursing, 18*(1), 13–20.

Lawton, M. P. (1982). Competence, environmental press, and the adaption of older people. In M. P. Lawton, P. G. Windley, & T. O. Byerts (Eds.), *Aging and the environment: Theoretical approaches* (pp. 33–59). New York: Springer Publishing Co.

Lawton, M. P., Windley, P. G., & Byerts, T. O., (Eds.). (1982). *Aging and the environment: Theoretical approaches*. New York: Springer Publishing Company.

Lucero, M. (1992, September). *Careplanning for dementia*. Paper presented at workshop, Wilsonville, OR. Sponsored by Oregon Assoc, of Homes for the Aged.

Mace, N. L. (1993). Observation of dementia specific care around the world. *American Journal of Alzheimer's Care and Related Disorders and Research, 11*(3), 1–8.

Managan, P. (1993, October). *Do old people come from outer space? Conflicts and dilemmas in clinical practice, legacy health care*. Paper presented at Portland, OR. Sponsored by Legacy Health Care System.

Mitchell-Pederson, L., Edmund, L., Fingerote, E., & Powell, C. (1986). Reducing reliance on physical restraints. *Today's Nursing Home, 7*(2), 40–46.

Moos, R. H., & Lemke, S. (1985). Assessing and improving socialecological settings. In E. Seidman (Ed.), *Handbook of Social Intervention*. Beverly Hills; CA: Sage Publications.

Rader, J. (1991). Modifying the environment to decrease use of restraints. *Journal of Gerontological Nursing, 17*(2), 9–13.

Restraint Minimization Project of New York Jewish Home & Hospital for Aged. (1993, February). How much does it cost? *Restraint Review, 3*.

Strumpf, N., & Evans, L. (1991). The ethical problems of prolonged physical restraint. *Journal of Gerontological Nursing, 17*(2), 27–30.

Tedros, N. (1992). Permanent assignment: The key to success. *Long Term Care Executive Network Newsletter, 1,* 6–7.

Williams, C. C. (1990, Fall). Long-term care and the human spirit. *Generations,* pp. 25–28.

Zgola, J. (1987). *Doing things.* Baltimore: Johns Hopkins University Press.

Zingmark, K., Norberg, A., & Sandman, P. O. (1993). Experience of at-homeness and homesickness in patients with Alzheimer's disease. *American Journal of Alzheimer's Care and Related Disorders and Research, 8*(3), 10–17.

Chapter 6

IDENTIFYING THE UNDERLYING CAUSE OF THE RESIDENT'S BEHAVIOR

Joanne Rader and Lynda Crandall

SYSTEMATIC DATA COLLECTION

The "detective" examines the resident's internal needs and the external environment to find the causes of behavioral symptoms. Sometimes a clear cause or causes can be identified, but often this is not possible, and it is necessary to make a "best guess" about why the resident is behaving in a particular way. In the past, nursing home staffs have often been frustrated in their efforts to identify causes. Much of this frustration, however, comes from several common shortcomings of the investigation process: failure to look at current medications as a potential source of excess disability, incomplete assessment of the external environment, impatience, incomplete or erratic data collection, reluctance to investigate physical problems and needs, inadequate assessment of the potential for pain and discomfort, and lack of adequate background information from resident or family.

Nursing home staffs have greatly improved their skills in assessing the internal needs of residents, and they are well attuned to physical causes of behavior changes. However, pain and discomfort are still often overlooked as a potential cause of agitation and restlessness. Many people with cognitive impairment lack the ability to tell the staff that they are in pain. The story of Mr. Terrance illustrates this well. Mr. Terrance, who had Alzheimer's disease, was admitted to the nursing home from the hospital for rehabilitation after he had a repair of his fractured hip. He had fallen in his foster home. He was also hard of hearing and wore bilateral hearing aids that had been lost in the hospital. He was able to respond to simple questions like, "How are you?" with "I am fine, thank you," but he could not engage in a lengthy conversation. He was admitted in the late morning and ate lunch in the facility. As the day wore on, he grew more and more restless. An observant CNA said to the evening nurse that she just had a hunch that something was not right with this gentleman, and she asked the nurse to take a look at him. The nurse discovered the cause of his increased restlessness; she found his hearing aid lodged in the back of his throat! It had been there long enough for the batteries to begin to corrode.

When we understand the symptoms of dementia, this situation is easily explained. First, Mr. Terrance's agnosia (inability to recognize objects) meant he would not recognize the hearing aid, and his hyperorality explains how it got into his mouth. Changes in his speech and language system explain why he was able to answer simple questions with social appropriateness yet was unable to express his distress in words. This example shows how dependent demented residents are on their caregivers to be good detectives who are willing to follow hunches, no matter how unusual they may seem.

If they are impatient, the staff may easily feel frustrated in their attempts to identify behavioral causes. If a person is engaging in a behavior that is potentially harmful and frightening to others, such as striking others, there is an understandable tendency to want an instant solution. However, the staff must be cautious, as one study has shown that much of the physically aggressive behaviors of persons with dementia result when staff members or others invade their personal space (Bridges-Parlet, Knopman, & Thompson, 1994). Yet physically aggressive behavior is a major reason for the overuse of psychoactive medications. A medication is given to control symptoms without investigating the underlying causes, and if it does not work quickly, there is a tendency to increase the dose or change the medication.

One way to try to counteract this tendency and still give staff members the sense that something is being done is to begin to collect data to identify underlying causes. The Health Care Financing Administration (HCFA) Interpretive Guidelines for Surveyors of Nursing Homes mandate that when certain psychoactive medications (antipsychotics, anxiolytics, and hypnotics) are used, there must be quantitative evidence that the medication is effective in reducing target symptoms. Good practice would suggest that collection of quantitative data should begin in the detective phase, not after the "carpenter" has already selected the "tool" of medication.

One method of data collection for both the detective and carpenter phases of intervention is the behavior monitoring chart described in Appendix A. The regulations do not state that data collection has to be continuous, and many facilities have found that continuous data collection over a period of months becomes rote and not truly reflective of behaviors. The best approach is to collect data on the frequency of the behavioral symptoms and the effectiveness of the intervention within a time frame that is reasonable for results to occur. For example, if the behavioral symptoms are striking at staff and other residents, swearing, and refusing to allow routine care and the best guess of the underlying cause—after other internal and external causes have been explored—is fearful delusions related to the dementia process, the intervention could be a low dose of an antipsychotic medication once a day. The staff should begin to document the target behaviors as part of the detective process, before intervening.

After initiating the use of medication (a carpenter's tool), it seems reasonable to collect data for at least 2 weeks, until the individual reaches steady state on the medication. If at that time there is good evidence that the medication has improved the behaviors, it would be reasonable to discontinue data collection and plan on reinitiating it 1–2 weeks prior to the quarterly review so that the medication can be reevaluated for efficacy, need for titration, and side effects. If after some time there is no evidence that the behaviors are continuing, that indicates either that the medication is effective or that the resident no longer needs the medication. The only way to sort that out, however, is to try a gradual, trial, slow dose reduction to see if the target behaviors reemerge at lower doses. The tendency of staff and physicians to not "rock the boat" if all is well is understandable. However, it is critical, particularly for persons with dementia who are receiving antipsychotics, to regularly reassess the need to continue because of the many potential side effects of these medications.

UTILIZING ALL AVAILABLE TEAM MEMBERS

The interdisciplinary team is crucial in identifying causes of behaviors. Involvement of the resident and family or significant other needs to be emphasized. They can provide key information about previous patterns and preferences. Without that information, a comprehensive approach to care is almost impossible, and any attempts to "manage" behaviors are likely to fail. Residents and families need guidance about their role in care planning. "Assessment and Care Planning," Appendix D, provides helpful information to residents and families.

There are other team members who are often not fully and skillfully utilized. In particular, the role of the physician is critical. There is great variation among physicians and among facilities in the quality of the medical care delivered and the extent of physician cooperation and coordination with other team members. The role of the facility medical director is also one that needs to be further defined and implemented.

Role of the Pharmacist

The pharmacist is another key team member who is frequently not fully utilized. The pharmacist's role includes both provider and consultant services. Provider services include dispensing drugs, maintaining a medication profile for clients, developing an audit system for controlled drugs, and maintaining the emergency drug supply. Consultant services are centered on drug-regimen review. These services may include communicating recommendations to physicians and staff, providing specific drug information, participating on committees, developing policies and procedures, providing in-service education, attending resident and family conferences, and developing quality assurance programs (Simonson, 1991).

There is great variation among facilities in terms of what the pharmacist does. In some facilities, for example, the pharmacist provides routine in-services for staff and families on psychoactive medications. In others, this never occurs.

If staff members feel that they need more services than they are currently receiving from the pharmacist, they should discuss it with the administration to see whether the problem rests with the pharmacist or whether the facility has not contracted with the pharmacist to provide those services. To expect nurses in long-term care to adequately monitor psychoactive medications without the support of consultants such as pharmacists and mental health professionals is imprudent.

Mental Health Assistance

One mechanism currently in place that provides some mental health assistance to facilities is the Preadmission Screening and Annual Resident Review (PASARR) process, which is federally mandated. The mechanisms for using this process when there is a serious behavioral symptom and the quality of the services vary from state to state. It may be useful to explore what services your state is offering through the PASARR process. When possible, the PASAAR evaluation process should be triggered before proposing to send a resident to an acute psychiatric inpatient unit for evaluation. Nursing homes are being asked to care for residents with increasingly difficult behavioral symptoms. It is useful for each facility to have in place a plan for managing behavioral emergencies. Appendix C, "Guidelines for Managing Behavioral Emergencies in the Nursing Home Setting," provides an outline of one recommended process.

COMMUNICATING WITH THE TEAM

The members of the treatment planning team are not always the same persons as those involved in the care conference. "Treatment team" is a term used to describe all persons contributing to the care planning process. They include the resident, the family, the physician, the staff of the facility, the case manager from Senior and Disabled Services or Mental Health, and the ombudsman, and perhaps others. The persons who attend the routine care conference may vary from meeting to meeting within a facility, or from facility to facility, but they commonly include the staff of the facility and the family. Given the inconsistency of attendance at actual care planning meetings, communication between the members of the entire treatment team is of paramount importance.

While staff at the facility participate in the care planning process, direct care staff (i.e., nurse's aides) and support services staff do not typically give formal input or attend resident care conferences. Direct care staff frequently have invaluable observations of behavior and good ideas about the origin of the behavior as well as strategies to address it. Further, these are often the persons expected to implement the plan of action designed in the care conference.

Commitment to a plan of care by the staff is enhanced when they individually and collectively feel ownership of the planning and design of the care. One way to achieve this is to invite input and actively use the information, observations, and ideas received. This can be done in a number of ways. It is obviously not necessary or practical to solicit ideas from every staff person on every identified problem for every resident. This type of approach may in fact be counterproductive. Welcoming input when a particular staff member offers it or asking for it when the team feels it prudent to seek additional information is a much more efficient use of everyone's time and energy. However, it is crucial to provide opportunities for input.

Oregon law requires that all nursing home residents be assigned a resident care manager (RCM). This is a registered nurse who is responsible and accountable for the resident's overall plan of care and for communicating it to involved parties. RCMs are required to have completed 30 continuing education hours or 3 college credit hours related to gerontology, rehabilitation or long-term care. In addition, they must have 3 college credit hours or 15 continuing credit hours pertinent to supervision. They generally facilitate the resident care conference. The role of the RCM has several advantages. It establishes who is responsible for seeing that all the elements of care come together in a way that makes sense for the resident. Having this one person responsible makes it easier to identify when someone is not doing her job well or when she is doing an exceptional job.

Information and ideas may come to the care conference in two ways:

1. Any staff person from any department, a family member, a physician, the resident, or any other member of the treatment team could be encouraged to direct questions, observations, or requests to the care conference team for discussion and problem solving. This could be done by a verbal statement to a member of the care conference team or by using a form designed for input to the team (see Figure 6.1).

2. Input could be solicited by the care conference team to broaden the data base to better understand a problem or to obtain help in figuring out solutions. This might be done in verbal exchanges between treatment team members and those attending care conference meetings or by using a form.

Having a policy for input to the care conference team and having forms are only a part of the process. A procedure to put the policy in practice may be necessary. One simple method is to post the schedule of care conferences and the list of residents to be reviewed at each meeting in several areas that are highly visible and accessible to staff (e.g., next to a time clock, in a prominent spot designated for this schedule in the nursing station, in the laundry department, in the kitchen, etc.). A supply of input forms can be left next to the schedule with clear, concise directions for using the forms. The forms can then be filled out by members of the treatment team who may not be planning to attend the care conference but may have information to aid in treatment and care planning. The forms are then returned to the RCM or a designee to be used by the care conference team in planning.

If the facility has implemented permanent assignments so that a certified nursing assistant on each shift has primary responsibility

Please fill out this form and return it to _____,
RCM/the care conference box. Answer whichever questions you find
pertinent. Thank you for taking the time.

To: The Care Conference Team
From: _____
Date: _____

Name of Resident: _____

1.   What question do you have regarding this resident?
     _____
     _____
     _____

2.   What behavior, action, symptom, problem or talk have you observed
     in the resident which you would like addressed with/for him/her?
     (Please be specific.)
     _____
     _____
     _____
     _____

3.   If it is a behavior you noted, when did you first notice it?
     _____

4.   What do you think might be the reason for the behavior?
     _____
     _____

5.   Why does this behavior concern you? (i.e., what impact does the
     behavior have on the resident or those around him/her?)
     _____
     _____

6.   Do you have intervention ideas (could be new ideas or
     interventions you/others have found to be helpful)?
     _____
     _____
     _____

7.   Other observations about this resident that you would like to
     communicate to the care conference team or that you would like
     discussed at the care conference.
     _____
     _____

8.   Would you like to attend the care conference? _____Yes _____ No

FIGURE 6.1

for a resident's care, it is particularly critical that their input is obtained for the conference in writing, through verbal communication with the nurse, or, ideally, by their presence at the conference. When the care conference staff wishes additional input, the RCM might send a memo to each department asking for the input by a particular date. The request can be disseminated to the various shifts through an intershift report, coordinated by the RCM and carried by the charge nurses.

Facilitating Communication with the Family and Family Participation in Care Planning

When a family places one of its family members in a long-term care setting, where most of the care is done by the staff of the facility, the family members often feel excluded from care planning. Some families may feel relief that they are no longer the sole providers and may wish to step back from the care planning temporarily or permanently. Many, however, wish to remain actively involved. Family collaboration with other treatment team members is key to excellent care. Some methods to encourage family input, communication, and participation are as follows:

1. The philosophy statement of the facility should include the family as an integral part of the team.
2. At the time of admission, family members should be presented an "orientation packet" that includes
   - a copy of the facility philosophy
   - a description of the care planning process and the role the family can play in that process
   - a description of how the facility recognizes staff for work well done (e.g., employee of the month, rewards, etc.)
   - a description of ongoing educational programs for staff and family members
   - a sample activity calendar
   - a list of facility services available (e.g., beauty shop, barber services, transportation, etc.) and how to access them

- names of management and key clinical staff, with telephone numbers
- visiting hours
- a list of community and facility resources (e.g., books, classes, support groups)
- volunteer opportunities and instructions on how to volunteer
- several free meal tickets so that they can join the resident for a meal or two
- information related to restraint-free care (see Appendix D, "The Freedom to Be Restraint Free: Information about Physical Restraints for Nursing Home Residents, Families & Friends")
- a questionnaire asking about the resident's history, usual daily activities, strengths, past behavioral difficulties, successful interventions, and questions the family may have about behavior or talk observed in the resident in the past or currently. This information should also be sought through an interview with the social worker or nurse manager. The written form, however, offers a way for the family to report information they may have omitted in the interview or were uncomfortable talking about.

3. Family members should be routinely invited to the care conference.

4. Family members should be invited to participate in care conferences through conference calls if they are unable to attend personally. This may permit someone who has no readily available transportation or someone who is unable to get away from work to have some input into care planning.

5. Care conference times and dates should be negotiated with the family to accommodate both the family and the staff.

6. Family members should be formally invited, by letter, to attend educational programs provided to the staff.

It might be useful to share "Assessment and Care Planning" (Appendix B), with residents and families. Facilities may wish to include this in their orientation packet or share it with family members prior to the family conference.

Facilitating Communication with the Physician and Participation in Care Planning

Physicians will be most responsive to your request for assistance in treating a resident's behavioral symptoms if you are prepared to discuss the situation in the way in which the physician is accustomed to discussing patients. This means using appropriate terminology to describe the behavioral symptoms, being specific about how the behavioral symptoms are distressing, rating the severity of the behavioral symptoms, describing the time course of the symptoms, and telling the physician what you or others have already done to deal with these symptoms. Communicating this information will improve the physician's decision making and decrease the chance of making a false diagnosis.

Most physicians are unable to routinely attend care conferences. This challenges the care conference team to diligently pursue input from the physician in planning care and to assure that the physician is kept informed of decisions made at the meetings. Keeping the physician apprised of meeting dates and times may be useful. (The care conference team may wish to save direct invitations for those very difficult cases that need the presence of the physician.) Input can take the form of written observations, suggestions, and the like from the physician. A form similar or identical to the one designed for staff input may prove useful for physicians as well. The form might be mailed to the physician a month in advance of the scheduled review, with a request for written input.

Communication between the nursing home and the physician is also crucial when the resident goes to the physician's office. This typically occurs after a nursing assessment is made of the particular complaint, symptom, or event. The information can be integrated into a summary note to the physician, or it may be relayed through a worksheet. The information sent to the physician serves two purposes:

1. It aids staff in assuring that the assessment and data are thorough and all indicated steps have been taken before the physician is called.
2. It provides the physician with all the important information.

In summary, it is crucial to include all team members in the process of identifying possible underlying causes of behavioral symptoms. If input is not sought from crucial members, it makes the process more difficult and frustrating. This in the long run takes more time and energy than systematically collecting the information when behaviors become problematic.

REFERENCES

Bridges-Parlet, S., Knopman, D., & Thompson, T. (1994). A descriptive study of physically aggressive behavior in dementia by direct observation. *Journal of American Geriatric Society*, 42, 192–197.

Simonson, W. (1991). *Consultant pharmacy practice*. Roche Laboratories.

Chapter 7

BALANCING THE BENEFIT AND BURDEN OF INTERVENTIONS

Joanne Rader

FROM THE RESIDENT'S PERSPECTIVE

In assessing the benefit and burden of potential interventions such as physical restraints and psychoactive medications, it is essential to take the resident's perspective. For example, Mr. Eaton, who was blind and had recently been admitted from home, had been receiving Valium for over 20 years. The staff was aware that Valium is a potentially unsafe drug for the elderly because of its long half-life. Therefore, they implemented very gradual dose reductions, and they observed that Mr. Eaton became much brighter and more interactive than when he had been on the larger doses. However, Mr. Eaton said he preferred the way he felt when he received the original dose. After several discussions with him and with his physician, in which he was informed about other, shorter-acting drugs that might be used and the potential negative characteristics of Valium, the staff honored his choice and returned him to the original dose of Valium. From his perspective, the benefits of how he felt on the Valium (and probably his need to be in control) outweighed what the staff perceived as the burdens. The staff planned to revisit this decision with him in the future and weigh with him again the possible benefits and burdens of his choice.

Mrs. Johnson further illustrates the importance of taking the resident's perspective. An 86-year-old woman living in her own home, she had severe rheumatoid arthritis and was becoming increasingly dependent on others for activities of daily living (ADLs); she was also experiencing more falls. Nevertheless, she stated quite clearly that she would rather lie on the floor of her own home waiting for someone to come and help her, than to be "safe" in a nursing home. Similarly, Mrs. Tuck, a 97-year-old nursing home resident with moderate dementia, had fallen numerous times and was currently recovering from a subdural hematoma. No treatable cause for the falls could be identified. The staff and the physician were fearful to such a point that the physician wrote as an order "restrain at all times; the next fall will be fatal." Mrs. Tuck preferred not to be restrained and stated quite clearly that she hated those things and was aware that she could fall and get hurt again but was willing to risk it. Clearly, at 97 years of age, something soon would be "fatal," and for her the benefits of freedom outweighed the risks even of death. Upon hearing her wishes, the staff discussed it further with the physician, who agreed to a gradual reduction in the use of the waist restraint. Staff began walking with her to improve her strength. She lived another 6 months completely restraint free, had several falls but no injuries falls and died quietly in her sleep.

It is of interest to note that health care providers rarely question the competence of individuals when they agree with our plans for them; competence is questioned only when they disagree. Yet, historically—as the case of physical restraints so clearly shows—the evidence indicates that professionals' choices and rationale may sometimes be terribly flawed.

In regard to physical restraints, it is helpful to think of the "cost" or "burden" of a device or intervention on a continuum, with the device becoming more costly or burdensome to the resident as it becomes more restrictive. Then, in using a device or intervention to address behavioral symptoms, the staff has an obligation to establish that the benefits outweigh the cost. Furthermore, the staff has an obligation to establish that the benefits for that level of restrictiveness are higher than they would be with an intervention at a lower level of restrictiveness *and* that the increased benefits outweigh the increased burden to the resident (see Figure 7.1).

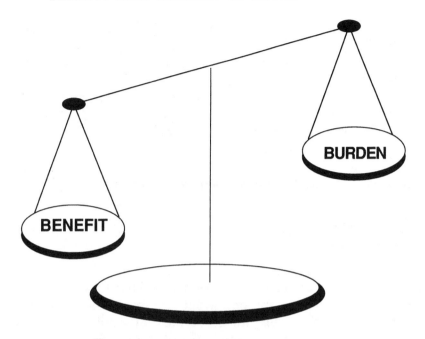

FIGURE 7.1   Benefit and burden scale.

For a resident who is unable to walk, the use of a soft waist tie-on device to provide support while in a wheelchair might allow the resident to propel himself and thus be more mobile. The benefit of increased mobility might be judged to outweigh the risk of abrasion or reduced circulation associated with the device. However, we would need to ask whether the same benefit (support to enhance mobility) could be obtained by a device that is less restrictive and therefore has a lower cost or burden to the resident (e.g., some type of specialized cushion or seating). It is also useful to recognize that an intervention to achieve one resident goal may serve as a barrier to achievement of another or related goal for the resident. For example, when a resident who has been restrained and using a standard sling-seat wheelchair is placed on a wedge cushion, to make him more comfortable and keep him from sliding, this often raises him 3–4 inches higher in the wheelchair. If he ambulates by using his feet in the wheelchair, and his feet no longer touch the ground, this intervention will have eliminated the use of a tie-on physical restraint, but it will still restrict his mobility. In this case, another step needs to be taken—to lower the wheelchair seat while continuing to use the wedge cushion so that the resident's feet will comfortably touch the floor.

When we rank goals, part of the "cost" of choosing higher-priority goals is relinquishment or postponement of goals ranked lower. For example, those in life-threatening situations sometimes benefit from devices that restrict mobility. Survival is ranked higher than the goal of mobility. That is to say, the cost of short term loss of mobility is outweighed by the benefit of living.

NEGOTIATING WITH THE RESIDENT AND FAMILY

It is impossible to understand the benefits and burdens of interventions for behavioral symptoms from the resident's perspective without discussing these with the resident or family (or a designated representative if the family is unable to participate). There is a tendency in our culture to leave elders and persons with disabilities out of decision making. We also assume that families will make decisions as the resident or patient would. This is not necessarily true. Often family members choose interventions for others that they would not want to endure themselves. Physical restraints and feeding tubes are examples.

As noted earlier, we often treat persons with dementia as if they lacked the capacity to make any decisions or to say no to interventions. In actuality, persons with dementia often have "windows of lucidity" in which they are capable of understanding information and the consequences of decisions. Further, while they may lack the capacity to comprehend the implications of some decisions, they may be quite capable of comprehending others. Also, while they may be incapable of comprehending the full consequence of behaviors such as attempting to pull out a feeding tube, if they consistently attempt to remove the tube, it is a clear indication that the tube is in some way a burden to them. If to maintain the tube you add the burden of restraining the arms, all that must be factored into the decision about benefit and burden, viewed as much as possible from the resident's perspective.

The federal guidelines require that informed consent be obtained from residents and families before using physical restraints or psychoactive medications. This is a departure from past practice. Formerly, facilities usually required a written release from responsibility when families asked that siderails or other physical restraints *not* be used. Now, just the opposite is required: the family's informed consent is necessary when restraints *are* used. If facilities propose the temporary use of a physical restraint, they are required to educate residents and families about the negative consequences of restraint use and propose a plan to move to less restrictive interventions (see Appendix D, "The Freedom to Be Restraint Free: Information about Physical Restraints for Nursing Home Residents, Families, and Friends").

The same holds true for psychoactive medications. Residents and families need to be informed about what the proposed benefits of the intervention are, as well as the burdens, such as side effects (see Appendix E, "Psychoactive Medication Information Sheets"). Families and residents therefore need access to information about these medications. The "Psychoactive Medication Information Sheets" provide basic information about the four major categories of psychoactive medications: antipsychotics, antidepressants, anxiolytics, and sedative/hypnotics. Reasons for use, names of commonly used drugs, and side effects are given for each category. Facilities may wish to share this material with residents and families as part of the informed consent process.

Facilities have reported that most residents and families are very supportive of the move to decrease the use of physical restraints and psychoactive medications. However, sometimes a family will object, and at times the family will insist on the use of a physical restraint, in spite of the team's assessment that it is not necessary and/or the resident's wish that it not be used. In many of these cases, the resident has some form of cognitive impairment, which complicates the issue of decision making. If a family objects to reducing restraint use, the facility should investigate to assure that the family is getting consistent messages from all team members.

Sometimes the staff on one shift may think restraints should be continued, and some may share their opinions and concerns with the family. This is like the facility shooting itself in the foot, and it serves only to confuse and distress the family. In 95%–98% of cases, if families are given current, consistent information on the negative effects of physical restraints and they participate in developing an alternative safety plan—viewed from the perspective of the resident—they are cooperative and pleased with the change in approach. Including the resident when possible and the family or designated representative in the negotiations for an acceptable safety plan is crucial and smart. If you are concerned about lawsuits (this concern sometimes drives practice more than resident wishes), include those most likely to sue in the decision-making process.

part III

"CUSTOMIZING" A SOLUTION

Chapter 8

OVERVIEW OF TYPES OF INTERVENTIONS

Joanne Rader

When looking for interventions to use in dealing with problematic situations, it is important to take a systematic approach. Facilities that take such an approach report a high degree of success in identifying underlying needs and reducing behaviors described as problematic without excessive use of physical restraints or psychoactive medications. First, as part of both the detective and carpenter roles, you look for physiological sources of excess disability, such as coexisting medical illnesses that have not been identified or are being inadequately treated and side effects from current medications.

If a physical problem is identified, then medical consultation or physiological interventions should be instituted. These may include such actions as medical evaluation, lab work, positioning, managing pain, stopping or starting a medication, changing the dose or time of a medication, and putting someone to bed when he is fatigued. Once you have ruled out the need for physiological or medical interventions, you now have four basic categories of "tools" or interventions to investigate for meeting the resident's identified needs: developing a supportive organizational environment, creating a supportive physical environment, using skillful psychosocial approaches, and using psychoactive medications appropriately (see Figure 3.1 in chapter 3). In most cases, the use of psychoactive medications should not be considered until all other categories of interventions have been explored and several options have been given adequate trials. In chapter 5 we discussed the need to explore the organizational environment for sources of unmet needs of residents, as part of the detective process. As a "carpenter," your job is to change aspects of the organizational environment, such as the belief or "rule" that all residents must have a bath or shower to be clean, and try alternatives like bed baths and evaluate the results. Moving the nursing home philosophy and practices from a hospital to a more homelike model is an often overlooked area for intervention. Yet adapting the existing philosophy, policies and procedures, staffing patterns, and structures of residents' days to better meet the needs of residents is essential in reducing behavioral symptoms and providing cost- and energy-efficient care. Changes may also need to be made in the physical environment, including noise level, lighting, furnishings, floor coverings, and equipment. The importance of providing comfortable, functional seating is discussed in detail in chapter 12.

Psychosocial interventions involve adapting and modifying the attitudes and approaches used by caregivers, improving staff communication skills, developing new strategies and techniques for responding to residents' emotional needs, and instituting appropriate activities and programs. Activities include formal activities, informal small groups, one-to-one activities, visiting, the general way in which the activities of daily living (eating, hygiene, and rest) are organized and carried out, and exercise. An important aspect of using skillful and creative psychosocial approaches is giving staff permission to be creative and practical in individualizing care.

Whatever area of intervention(s) you choose first, establish a good data base, using some form of behavior monitoring. One form of monitoring, along with instructions for its use, is found in Appendix A. Then, after choosing an intervention, allow sufficient time to carry out the intervention(s), and take the intervention to the "max." For example, if you think that a person's yelling during care activities is caused by pain from arthritis, then you should ensure that antiinflammatory arthritis drugs are given routinely in sufficient amounts (unless contraindicated by side effects, etc.) to be effective before you decide that the drug is not helping or that arthritic pain is not the problem. This is critical to truly evaluate the outcome. Too often staff are in such a hurry to eliminate the perceived problem that they jump from intervention to intervention without giving each a complete trial. Then they are more likely to feel frustrated, hopeless, and defeated.

Chapter 9

ORGANIZATIONAL CHANGES

Joanne Rader

Chapter 5 discussed organizational issues that need to be addressed as part of the detective process. This chapter describes the development of a supportive organizational environment as an intervention. Two examples are used to illustrate the process: the reduction of physical restraints and the reduction of psychoactive medications.

ORGANIZATIONAL CHANGE RELATED TO PHYSICAL RESTRAINTS

It is important to remember that eliminating the use of physical restraints in long-term care is a dramatic shift in practice that requires time, support, education, and successful experiences in order to take hold. Making the transition to a restraint-free facility is a process that must occur on several levels.

Get Administrative Support

To begin the process of eliminating restraints, it is important to get support and commitment from individuals who have decision-making and action authority. Administrators must agree to support a restraint-reduction program. This is perhaps a less difficult task now in nursing homes because of the mandate for change in the 1990 Health Care Financing Administration (HCFA) guidelines for state surveyors.

Form a Committee or Task Force

You may find it useful to form a steering committee to study the literature, talk with people from restraint-free facilities, and develop a policy or philosophy statement to take to the facility staff and board of directors if that is appropriate. The steering committee will need to assess the strengths and weaknesses of the facility in relation to restraint reduction (number of secured and unsecured doors, available equipment, type and frequency of activities, etc.). The committee can also decide on the best way to inform physicians, families, residents, and staff about the planned change in practice. In larger facilities, a formal committee may be formed and meet weekly or monthly. In smaller facilities, the group may be more informal and meet over coffee break. There is no one "right" way.

Appoint a Coordinator

Appointing a project coordinator or facility resource person is helpful. A coordinator can serve as a cheerleader and an information and idea source. Because there are many pressures on facility staff, it is important that someone is designated to *keep* restraint reduction a priority. Having at least one individual in the facility who is committed to eliminating restraints yet realistic about current resources and skills is crucial. This person can guide and provide support to others. Those facilities that have been most successful in reducing restraint use have had such an individual on staff. Without that type of commitment and leadership, the process will falter.

Evaluate Forms

Do the current forms perpetuate old attitudes? For example, do the admission orders have a space for the physician to check if he or she wishes restraints? Since restraints are to be the exception rather than the rule, this is no longer appropriate and may mislead the physician.

Gain Staff Commitment

Once support and direction from the top have been established, it is important to get "grass-roots" support from the nursing staff and other line staff. Initially, there may be fear, skepticism, and even anger. These are healthy reactions to change and need to be acknowledged and addressed. The staff needs to be assured that there will be a new way of looking at falls, risks, and resident rights, and they will be supported in their efforts to change.

The best way for the staff to learn new attitudes and approaches is through role modeling by supervisors, advocates, families, and coworkers. A blaming, judgmental response is harsh and unproductive. A supportive, instructive response frees staff members to view their role and approaches in new ways and allows the magic of caring to flow to residents.

For example, a nurse overheard a new certified nursing assistant (CNA) raising her voice in anger and telling a resident, "Come to the bathroom now! I have others to care for." The resident became agitated and resistive. The nurse moved into the situation and spoke softly, with a warm smile, to the resident and gave one-step commands such as "stand," "walk with me," and so on. The nurse instructed the CNA to come along to the bathroom. After the resident's needs were met, she explained to the CNA the specific things she did that elicited cooperation from the resident, and told the CNA to be sure to seek her help in the future if she had difficulties.

If a staff member's refusal to change his or her thinking and practices becomes intolerable—and education, support, and consultation have been provided—action needs to be taken. Administrators need to clarify that the staff member's out-of-date, controlling, harsh approach to care will not be tolerated and, if continued, will be grounds for reprimand or dismissal.

Evaluate Current Practices

Track the number of residents who currently have physical restraints (including siderails that are restraints [see chapter 11]). Also track falls and injuries related to falls (chapter 11). Evaluate the facility's current statistics on falls and injuries. This establishes a baseline from which to measure progress and serves as a quality assurance check and feedback mechanism for staff. Posting each unit's progress toward restraint-free care on a monthly basis can be useful and encouraging.

Train Staff

For a restraint-reduction program to be effective, it is essential to orient staff to its importance. It is equally important to continue educating and supporting them throughout the implementation process and on an ongoing basis. Many facilities use the care planning conference as a way to educate staff and families about the restraint-reduction process. Topics for training and education sessions include these:

- A review of negative effects and burdens of restraints
- The resident assessment process and tools
- Alternative interventions
- Fall prevention and assessment
- Ways to stimulate creative problem solving
- The importance of residents' rights.

A basic building block upon which most other interventions rely is training in how to communicate with confused residents (see chapter 13).

Orient Physicians

Send the physicians a letter to explain the changes in practice and regulations. Figure 9.1 is a sample letter. It is helpful to enclose copies of articles written by physicians that support the need for this change. Useful articles include Marks, W. (1992) "Physical

Dear Dr:
   We are writing to tell you about an exciting change in practice that will affect the care of your patients in our nursing home. New information about care practices in some European countries and in selected facilities in the United States, and some recent studies have raised serious questions about the practice of using physical restraints routinely. As a result, the nursing home reform act (OBRA) effective October 1, 1991, requires these significant changes:

1. Prn orders for physical restraints will no longer be accepted.
2. Restraints may be used only after less restrictive means have been attempted and failed, or temporarily if there is a life-threatening situation.
3. Restraint orders must specify the type of restraint, the reason it is used, the circumstances under which it is to be used and the length of time it is to be used.
4. The resident, family member, or legal guardian must give consent for its use.

As a facility, we support these changes and ask for your assistance in making them. We are working to educate our staff and develop more individualized care approaches that address safety needs without the use of restraints. Enclosed are the Health Care Financing Administration (HCFA) Interpretive Guidelines related to physical restraints, along with several articles that support this change in practice. Please feel free to call if you have questions.

Sincerely,

Administration

Director of Nursing

Figure 9.1   Sample letter to physicians

Restraints in the Practice of Medicine," and Miles, S. H., and Irvine, P. (1992) "Deaths Caused by Physical Restraints." These articles illustrate the clinical reasons for the change. You would also want to include "The Freedom to Be Restraint-Free: Information about Physical Restraints for Nursing Home Residents, Families, and Friends" (Appendix D). The person organizing the restraint-reduction program also could meet with a group of physicians or speak with them individually. The appropriate process will vary by facility and physician.

Start with Easiest Residents First

It is important to begin restraint reduction and elimination in a planned systematic way. Determine which resident seems to have the least safety risks. Select one or two in this group and begin a gradual progressive reduction. You may remove the restraints for

1–2 hours per shift and place the resident within view while staff assess how the person responds. You may also chose to concentrate on one area or unit at a time. The important thing is that continued progressive reduction occur.

Prevent Backsliding

It is important for facilities to be aware of the possibility of back-sliding. Several facilities in Oregon have reported that following an initial campaign and push to decrease the use of restraints, there were dramatic reductions in use. However, if there was not some-one present in the environment who could act as a resource and also as promoter of change, the use of restraints began to increase again. This may occur for a variety of reasons. First, the change in practice is still new and the staff often resorts to old patterns or solutions unless challenged. Second, restraints may be too avail-able to the staff or staff members may not be evaluating their use routinely.

Several strategies can prevent backsliding once significant pro-gress has been made:

- Do not leave attached tie-on restraints on the units where they are easily accessible to the staff.
- If restraints are on the units, make a policy that they should be put on only by the nurse and that the resident should be reevaluated at least at each shift, to determine if his condition still warrants restraint.
- Permit only the DNS or designated person to give out restraints.
- Have a policy by which the administrator or DNS must be called before restraints are used.

These strategies may sound rather extreme, but facilities commit-ted to changing the practice have found them very successful.

More and more facilities are eliminating restraints or reducing their use to below 5%, illustrating that it can be done safely with current staffing levels and minimal expenditures for new equipment (Restraint Minimization Project, 1993). Thus, it is becoming more difficult to justify the continued use of restraints. In a sense, the staff needs to begin to think of physical restraints as an obsolete practice, much as we have come to think of the use of heat lamps for decubitus ulcers as obsolete. If a nurse continued to use heat lamps, she would be told by her colleagues and administrators that she would not be permitted to continue an out-of-date practice. Restraints are quickly becoming as out of date as heat lamps.

Consultation

Another useful organizational strategy is to require consultation with another professional before a restraint is initiated. This may be the physical or occupational therapist, another nurse, or an expert at another facility. It is critical that we break away from the old view that restraints are acceptable practice. Indeed, it is helpful to look at restraint use as a strategy that contains so much potential for hazardous side effects that, like hanging a unit of blood, it requires a double check by another professional to assure that the highest and safest standards of practice are applied.

Supervisors and administrators can play an important role in reducing restraint use and bringing out true caring for residents in direct caregivers by

- creating an environment that encourages staff to develop relationships with residents
- creating an environment that minimizes stress
- creating an environment that does not demand that residents adapt to the facility's routines
- defining the caregiver's job as helping residents meet both their expressed and unexpressed needs, not as completing a series of tasks during the shift
- providing support and encouragement to staff.

The rewards for staff who care for nursing home residents do not come from meeting administrative expectations or state or federal regulations. The joy for staff comes from knowing that what they do and how they do it makes a difference in the life of another human being. That is the source of staff motivation and satisfaction. The staff's caring for residents can be nurtured by

- organizing the daily work to facilitate staff efforts
- ensuring that administrators, regulators, family, and advocates treat staff in supportive ways
- providing education, consultation, and resources

When the administration creates a caring environment for caregivers as well as for residents, then caregivers are better able to take on the magician's role as the first step toward understanding behavioral symptoms, the detective's role in determining their causes, and the carpenter's role in developing interventions.

ORGANIZATIONAL CHANGE RELATED TO MEDICATIONS

Changing the way we use psychoactive medications also requires organizational strategies. Because, in the past, staff members lacked the tools to cope with behavioral symptoms, they often requested the use of medications prematurely and inappropriately. Many of the strategies for changing restraint use mentioned above are applicable to medication use. Specific strategies to improve staff skills include establishing a committee or group to brainstorm difficult behavioral symptoms, establishing a psychoactive medication review committee, expanding the role of the clinical pharmacist, using mental health consultation, providing resource books, sending key nurses to classes and workshops on the use of psychoactive medications and coping with behaviors, and educating physicians about the federal guidelines and the need for them to write a justification if they wish to prescribe outside the guidelines.

Very few people in long-term care facilities enjoy the thought of another committee or meeting; however, when a major change in practice is needed or required, it is often the most time- and cost-effective and the most supportive way to implement the change. Numerous facilities have established behavioral symptom groups or committees that brainstorm how to resolve difficult situations without the use of physical restraints or medications. One format involves discussing general case studies. With this format you can use one committee to discuss both physical and chemical restraints.

Another approach is to take a category of psychoactive medications and review the characteristics of the class of drugs, as well as the side effects and efficacy profiles of each drug, and then discuss a case related to that specific category at each meeting. Committees may be "ad hoc" so that when the facility eliminates the use of restraints and significantly reduces medications, they can be disbanded. Or the facility may find such a committee a useful forum for developing creative solutions for difficult behaviors and continue it. You may wish to incorporate the committee work into care conferences and quarterly reviews.

It is important to try to have a clinical pharmacist and/or mental health professional attend the meetings or be readily available for consultation. The judicious, skillful use of psychoactive medications is complex. Nurses, social workers, and physicians in nursing homes are usually generalists. To ask them to be "experts" and not provide them with expert consultation and advice is unwise and adds to the high cost of poor care.

Access to information about medications such as half-life, time of onset, and peak action is essential. Therefore, the team needs to have adequate resource books available. The *Physician's Desk Reference* is commonly found on nursing units, yet it is rarely the best source of information. Consult with the pharmacist for a list of books that she would recommend. A pharmacology book designed for nurses is often useful.

REFERENCES

Marks, W. (1992). Physical restraints in the practice of medicine: Current concepts. *Archives of Internal Medicine, 152,* 2203–2206.

Miles, S. H., & Irvine, P. (1992). Deaths caused by physical restraints. *The Gerontologist*, 32(6), 762–766.

Restraint Minimization Project, Jewish Home and Hospital for the Aged, New York. (1993, February). "How much does it cost?" *Restraint Review*, p. 6.

Chapter 10

CREATING A SUPPORTIVE ENVIRONMENT FOR ELIMINATING RESTRAINTS

Joanne Rader

This chapter focuses on interventions for creating a nursing home environment that is free from the use of physical restraints and uses other restrictive interventions only for limited, goal-directed periods. Many of the interventions described here adapt the physical environment. The psychosocial environment is also addressed.

It is important to understand the current definition of a physical restraint. The definitions of physical restraints that appear in the April 1992 Health Care Financing Administration (HCFA) Interpretive Guidelines (483.13 Ftag 221) are as follows: "physical restraints" are any manual method or physical or mechanical device, material, or equipment attached or adjacent to the resident's body that the individual cannot remove easily and that restricts freedom of movement or normal access to one's body.

Physical restraints include, but are not limited to, leg restraints, arm restraints, hand mitts, soft ties or vests, and wheelchair safety bars. Also included as restraints are facility practices that meet the definition of a restraint, such as tucking in a sheet so tightly that a bedbound resident cannot move, bedrails, chairs that prevent rising, or placing a wheelchair-bound resident so close to a wall that the wall prevents the resident from rising. (See also 42 CRF

483.25(h), *Accidents*, for bedrails.) Wrist bands or devices on clothing that trigger electronic alarms to warn staff that a resident is leaving a room do not, in and of themselves, restrict freedom of movement and should not be considered as restraints.

"Chemical restraints" means a psychopharmacologic drug that is used for discipline or convenience and is not required to treat medical symptoms.

These definitions reflect the purpose of the new regulation, which is to enhance the resident's freedom of movement and normal access to the body. Furthermore, the definition of physical restraints identifies some of the devices that have frequently been used to restrict freedom of movement and normal access to the body.

Although this list of devices can serve as a "red flag," it is incomplete and likely to be revised over time as we gain more experience in implementing the desired changes in practice. In addition, it is misleading to define "restraints" only in terms of a device, without taking into consideration the effect of the device on the individual resident.

When facilities are described as being restraint-free or working toward that as a goal, generally this means they are

1. eliminating the use of all tie-on physical restraints
2. eliminating the use of siderails that prevent residents from getting out of bed if they wish
3. using other devices for the purpose of restricting mobility such as reclining chairs and lap trays only as a last resort, for specific behaviors and for short periods.

When any device is used to restrict mobility, it is defined by HCFA as a physical restraints and requires a physician's order.

A reclining chair used to bring a semicomatose resident out of his room and provide a position change is not a restraint. The same chair used to prevent a demented, pacing resident from rising so as to provide a brief period of rest and improve balance when he is fatigued is a physical restraint. This would require a physician's order such as "recliner for 15–30 minutes until balance improves."

If staff members use this chair for prolonged periods, to prevent wandering, they will be using it inappropriately and without proper authorization.

The focus should be on modifying our practice to comply with the *intent* of the regulations. The following guidelines can assist with this.

First, examine *all* devices, material, and equipment for their *potential to restrict mobility*, whether or not they are on a list generated by HCFA.

Second, consider all devices, material, and equipment for their *potential to enhance mobility*.

Third, conduct an individual assessment prior to using any device that has the potential to restrict or withholding any device that has the potential to enhance mobility.

Fourth, specify the *goal* that suggests the need for a device/ intervention having the potential to restrict freedom of movement or normal access to the body. Goals can generally be put into one of three categories: (1) to promote safety, (2) to facilitate short-term therapeutic treatment, or (3) to provide support needed to enhance mobility.

Fifth, select the least restrictive or potentially least harmful device or intervention that will meet the established goal. Strive to decrease the length of time it is in use.

Sixth, carefully weigh the burden of using that device or intervention (if it has the potential to restrict mobility) against the benefit of meeting the established goal.

Seventh, seek consensus around the goal and use of the device to obtain the goal (consult the resident and/or family, staff, and physician).

In following these guidelines, it is useful to think about devices/ interventions as existing on a continuum of restrictiveness. Any device that the resident cannot remove is more restrictive than one that the resident can remove. In general, adjacent devices would be considered less restrictive than attached devices. Environmental modifications would be considered less restrictive than either adjacent or attached devices. If a restrictive device is currently being used for a resident, we can ask if a less restrictive device would meet the goal. If a new restrictive device is being considered, we can choose one of the least restrictive to accomplish the goal. Figure 10.1 identifies some of the more commonly used adjacent and attached devices and provides a continuum of restrictiveness as a guide for choosing the "least" restrictive device. In following this guide, it is also helpful to think of the cost or burden of the device/intervention as also existing on a continuum, with the device being more costly or burdensome to the resident as it becomes more restrictive. Although it is usually desirable to move to no devices or to the less restricted devices listed in Figure 10.1, it should not be an automatic move without considering the effect on the individual withholding certain devices with some residents may decrease their function, and, therefore, be more restrictive. All devices and interventions must be assessed from the resident's perspective to determine how it affects function or freedom. A side rail left up on one side of the bed, may enhance some residents' bed mobility.

In the past, we considered tie-on physical restraints and siderails to have only benefits. We were unaware of their many potential negative physical consequences, and we ignored the tremendous emotional burden they created for the individual. It is time to incorporate this new understanding into our decision making.

DEGREE OF RESTRICTIVENESS

Least	⟶	Most
	Adjacent devices	**Attached devices**
Over bed table	Recliner/tilted chair which prevents the individual from rising	Pelvic
Lap board		Vest-Torso
Wheelchair brake resident is unable to remove	Gerichair with locked tray table which prevents the individual from rising	Waist
Wedge cushions	Seat belt which cannot be removed by resident	Mitt
		Leg
Support pillows and devices	Side rails that prevent the individual from getting out of bed	Wrist
		Ankle

* While it is desirable to move to less restrictive devices or no devices, this should not be an automatic move made without considering the effect on the individual. Withholding certain devices from some residents may decrease their function and, therefore, be more restrictive.

FIGURE 10.1 Devices that may restrict movement.

Chapter 11 addresses issues of siderail use in depth and provides a new look at an old practice.

We now know that physical restraints, including siderails (see Chapter 11), have many negative consequences and that their efficacy in avoiding the reasons for restraint use is not supported by the literature. However, the staff in nursing homes needs considerable information and support to make the transition to restraint-free care. The following list of useful interventions is meant to stimulate creativity, identify problems and their resolutions, and help in this transition.

USEFUL INTERVENTIONS

The list of useful interventions is organized around the behaviors that most commonly lead to the use of restraints, and it gives types of interventions to explore with each behavior. Physical and medical interventions such as ruling out diseases or other medical problems, treating these problems when possible, toileting routinely, and managing pain are so extensive and individualized that this list does not include them. The assumption is that staff will consider those types of interventions *before* looking at environmental, psychosocial, and activity approaches. In most cases, the medical-physical evaluation should precede the use of other interventions.

Information on where to obtain specific devices mentioned in this list can be found in the resource list in Appendix F.

Interventions Related to Falling

Behavior: Leaning or Sliding in Chair

Environmental Interventions

- Have a wheelchair or seating assessment done by a physical therapist or occupational therapist.
- Adjust the wheelchair back and seat to create a slight tilt back and wedge (from L to V).
- Try a type of specialized cushion.

- Create a nonslip surface by using a variety of products: Dycem, Scoot-gard, nonslip rug backing, Rubbermaid shower or bath decals, or bath mat. (The cost of these products varies, and often the cheapest works fine.)
- Try a comfortable reclining chair.
- Try types of position-change alarms: Ambularm, Chair Sentinel, Posey Sitter, Tabs, Window Alarm (guidelines for the use of alerting devices are given in Table 10.1).
- Try overbed table, lap boards.
- Try a seat belt that the resident is able to remove.
- Try formed foam pads.
- Try a solid seat insert.
- Adapt a recliner or wheelchair with an extended, padded backrest (this can be fabricated or purchased).

Sometimes a combination of these approaches is necessary to solve the problem. For example, you may need to use a solid seat wedge insert placed in the wheelchair over a Scoot-Gard pad.

Psychosocial/Activity Interventions

- Place the resident within view of the staff.
- Respond to toileting and comfort needs.
- Put the resident to bed when she is fatigued.
- Place diversional activities in front of the person.

Behavior: Unsafe Mobility

Environmental Interventions

- Have a seating and mobility assessment done by the physical therapist or occupational therapist.
- Use position-change alarms: Ambularm, Chair Sentinel, Posey Sitter, Tabs, Window Alarm (see Figure 10.2).
- Try pressure-change alarms: Bedcheck, Code Alert, Posey Sitter, Virgil 88 (guidelines for use of these alarms are given in Figure 10.2).
- Attach a call light to the resident's gown.

Table 10.1   Guidelines for Assessing Use of Alerting Devices

Alerting devices have been used in many nursing facilities as part of a safety plan when decreasing or eliminating physical restraints. These types of devices sound an alarm when the resident changes position, lifts his or her weight off a bed or chair, or exceeds the limits of a cord attached from the resident to the chair or bed. One way these devices have been used is as a substitute call light for residents who are unsafely mobile and cognitively unable to use the call light. When a staff member hears the alarm, it is a message to assist the resident, rather than to simply tell the resident to sit down—a command that may have the effect of reducing, rather then enhancing, the resident's mobility.

Alerting devices may be used routinely for specified times during the day or until balance or endurance improve. Residents and families need to be clearly informed that these devices in no way can assure safety but are merely one part of a safety plan, and there may be times when the alarm will not work (the resident removes it or the alarm fails to sound or is slow to do so). It is not fail-safe, but merely a tool intended to increase the resident's safety. Position- and pressure-change alarms may restrict freedom and privacy to a degree, so ethically they must be used only after careful assessment and discussions with the resident and/or family.

These devices have been found to be particularly useful for the types of person listed below and for those with combinations of these problems:

1. Mild forgetfulness or impaired judgment and restricted weight-bearing status following orthopedic surgery
2. Impaired mobility, judgment, and balance following a stroke
3. Dementia and an unreliable or unsteady gait
4. Ambulation to the bathroom at night by oneself but with incontinence along the way or periods of transient dizziness
5. Poor balance or unsteady gait attempting to get out of bed without assistance
6. A history of frequent falls

Before initiating use of a position or pressure-change alarm, it is helpful to take the following steps:

1. Conduct a mobility assessment (see Chapter 11).
2. If the resident passes such an assessment, it is probably not appropriate to use a position-change alarm.

(continued)

Table 10.1 *Continued*

3. If mobility problems are found to exist, administer a more detailed gait evaluation. An example is the Tinetti Balance and Gait Evaluation (see Figure 11.1). Contact the resident's physician to share the results of the evaluation and explore the possibility of seeking an underlying cause or requesting a physical therapy consult for gait and/or balance training.
4. Discuss the use of the device with the resident and/or family.

After initiating use of the device, consider the following:

1. If the resident removes it frequently or tries to, it may not be the best intervention, and a different safety plan should be developed. Frequent attempts at removal may indicate that the device is a burden on the resident.
2. Use of the device should be continually reevaluated (at least every 3 months). If indicated and following discussion with resident and/or family, conduct a 3-day trial without the device, evaluating the results from the resident's perspective. During those trial days, each shift should document the resident's responses.
3. If the resident is no longer mobile or has ceased attempting to stand and the situation seems likely to remain unchanged, the device should be removed.

Costs of alerting devices vary greatly. Alarms designed specifically for resident use may cost up to $150 to $200 each. Some facilities have adapted window and burglar alarms for this purpose by attaching the cord-pull alarms in various ways to wheelchairs or beds; the cost of these devices is in the $10–$30 range.

Finally, there are as yet no studies that show that alarm devices alone prevent falls or injury. Since our culture tends to be overprotective of the elderly and to seek solutions in technology, it is easy to overrely on these devices instead of seeking the underlying causes of falls and instability. When considering use of a device, it is important to ask, "Is this to increase the resident's safety or to make the staff feel more secure?" A number of facilities report that they found these devices initially useful as they were reducing restraint use, but over time, as their assessment and intervention skills increased, they no longer felt the need to use the devices.

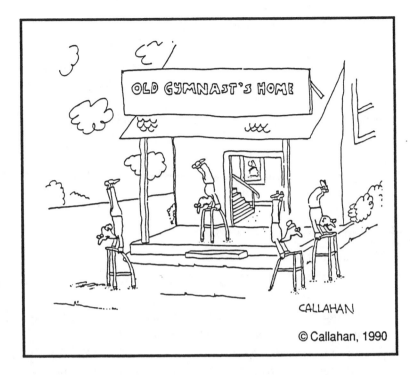

OLD GYMNAST'S HOME

CALLAHAN

© Callahan, 1990

- Attach bells on lap robe, blanket, or siderails.
- Place the bed lower to the floor to allow the resident's feet to touch the floor.
- Check for appropriate shoes (a shuffling gait may require a sole that can slide).
- Remove unnecessary objects that might cause the resident to trip.
- Assess the use of furniture with wheels and furniture that is unstable; remove if it is used by the resident for support.
- Provide adequate lighting.
- Monitor activity in the resident's room with a nursery intercom walkie-talkie (Mattell, Fisher-Price, etc.).
- Provide supportive, assistive devices and keep them within reach of the resident (these include glasses and hearing aids if appropriate).

- Place a commode at the bedside.
- Assess the use of various walkers—Chariot, Ultimate, Able.
- Use a nonslip bath mat or rug at the bedside or commode to improve traction (this is particularly helpful if the person is prone to slipping in his own urine).
- Try nonskid-bottom socks: You can purchase these or make them by using plain socks and rubberized fabric-decorating pens to put nonslip lines on sock bottoms.
- Try exit alarms that emit a beep when crossed (Radio Shack or Alert Care Exit Alarm).

Psychosocial/Activity Interventions

- Anticipate the resident's needs.
- Learn the resident's past patterns and coping styles, toileting schedule, and habits.
- Use balance boards or exercise pedals while the resident is seated to improve balance and endurance.
- Provide frequent accompanied walks; include the family and show them how to assist the resident if appropriate.
- Use naturally occurring opportunities to assist residents to walk to and from the bed, bath, and meals instead of using a wheelchair.
- Develop formal, routine exercise programs geared to the residents' level of participation.

Behavior: Standing Unsteadily but Generally Lacking Ability to Walk

Environmental Interventions

- Have a seating and mobility assessment done by the physical therapist or occupational therapist.
- Place the resident's bed in a low position so that his center of gravity and bend of the knees make it hard for the individual to come to a standing position.
- Try a Chariot or Ultimate Walker.

Psychosocial/Activity Interventions

- Offer adequate stimulation and small group gatherings.
- Offer the resident things to fiddle with and/or look at.
- Try giving the resident an apron, with dust rags and other objects in the pockets.
- Try dolls or stuffed toys to provide comfort or diversion.

Behavior: Climbing or Falling Out of Bed

Interventions for Residents Who Are Going over the Siderails

- Have a seating and mobility assessment done by a physical therapist or occupational therapist.
- Put the rail down.
- Place the resident in a low bed (guidelines for the use of low beds are given in Table 10.2).
- Place the resident's mattress on a futon frame.
- Place the mattress on the floor (check the fire regulations).
- Pin a call light to the resident's clothes.
- Use three-quarter- or half-length siderails to prevent rolling out of bed.
- Use a position-change alarm: Ambularm, Tabs, Radio Shack.
- Use a pressure-change alarm: Bed Check, Posey Sitter, Code Alert, Vigil 88.
- Monitor activity in the resident's room with a nursery intercom walkie-talkie.
- Try sitting with the person and soothing him with talk or touch to help him fall asleep or at least calm down.
- Get the person out of bed, even at night; provide food and drink.
- Try relaxation tapes or music.
- Identify activities that the resident finds pleasurable.
- Bring the resident into a lighted area.
- Try bringing the resident's bed near the nurses' station.

- Place a pillow or rolled blanket under the mattress to create a lip at the edge.
- Place furniture or a chair against the bed; be sure the furniture is not unstable if the person is likely to use it for support.
- Place a foam egg crate mattress covered with a sheet next to a low bed.
- Try a triangular foam wedge or rolled-up egg crate mattress tucked next to the rail to form a "cradle."
- Monitor activity in the resident's room with a nursery intercom walkie-talkie.

Falls prevention is discussed in more detail in chapter 11.

Table 10.2   Guidelines for Placing Mattress on Low Platform

For many residents, being restricted in bed by a tie-on restraint or siderail is a source of distress and agitation, yet they are at risk if they attempt to get out of bed on their own. Many lack the memory or judgment to call for assistance.

A successful safety intervention is placing the resident's mattress on a low platform (14–18 inches from floor). This low platform may be a Hollywood-style metal bed frame with a sheet of plywood cut to fit in the frame or a wooden futon frame to support the mattress from a regular bed. Metal frames can often be obtained at secondhand stores. Be sure to round off the corners of the plywood platform so that they do not extend and create a hazard for residents and staff. It costs approximately $30 to put the metal frame and plywood together; the cost of futon frames varies.

This platform allows the resident to be restraint-free when in bed. Sometimes lowering the bed allows the resident better traction because the feet touch the floor. Sometimes the bed may need to be lowered so that he/she is unable to come to a standing position from which he/she would be at risk for a fall. Another reason to lower the bed is to shorten the distance the resident would fall if he/she were to roll out of bed. If the floor is vinyl linoleum and the resident is still able to stand or walk, you may wish to place a rubber backed, beveled edged rug next to the bed to improve traction. This is also a useful intervention if the resident is incontinent of urine and is at risk for slipping, because the rug absorbs the urine and ensures better footing. If the resident is no longer able to stand but is at risk for rolling out of bed, in addition to lowering

(continued)

Table 10.2 *Continued*

the bed you may "bring the floor up" and cushion the floor by placing a thick mat or foam egg crate mattress by the side of the bed. This can be slipped under the bed or rolled up out of the way when the resident is not in bed.

Here are some useful questions to ask when considering lowering the bed.

1. Have all possible reasons why the person is at risk for falls been evaluated (medications, illness)?
2. Would the bed create other risks if positioned low (e.g., following hip surgery flexion > 90°)?
3. Have all the other ways to minimize risk that could be used in place of or in addition to placing the bed lower been considered i.e., would the use of a position-change alarm increase the safety margin? This may be a useful adjunct when the bed is on a low platform.
4. Are there any additional interventions necessary to increase the resident's comfort and safety (e.g., rug or mat next to bed)?
5. Are the resident's weight, weight-bearing status, and care needs such that a low bed will not place an undue burden on the nursing staff?
6. Is any in-service required for the staff so that they will be aware of how to care for and transfer the resident in the safest way possible, for both resident and staff?
7. Has the risk-benefit ratio been weighed with the resident and/or family?
8. Have the resident and family been consulted and have they agreed to this safety intervention?
9. Has the assessment and intervention selection process been documented in the chart?
10. Are there other safety factors to consider in the room with the bed on the floor (e.g., need to put safety plugs in outlets or need to move bedside stand to prevent patient from pulling up on it)?

If these questions have been addressed and the assessment indicates that the resident would benefit from placing the bed nearer to the floor, the nurse should notify the appropriate staff member, who will obtain the platform and lower the bed. Generally, staff members have found that it is easier to utilize the low bed when it is on wheels.

(continued)

Table 10.2 *Continued*

Caution: This intervention may not be appropriate for residents if they are very heavy; require frequent, complex care in bed; and/or are unable to bear weight.

Residents with some or all of these characteristics may pose too great a risk of staff injury. This possibility would need to be included in the assessment process.

Keep in mind that nurse's aides are very clever and creative and can find ways to care for residents in low beds that are safe and convenient for them. For example, the aide might get the resident up in a wheelchair and wash him/her at the sink rather then doing so in the low bed.

For the few residents who could be restraint-free with a low bed, but for whom the low bed is not appropriate because of their weight or heavy care needs, the facility should purchase new high-low beds that have the capacity to be lowered for safety and raised when care is given. *It is not appropriate to restrain a person in bed because the proper bed is not available.*

Some local fire marshals have concerns about beds without wheels. If there is an objection, you may wish to contact the state fire marshal and request a waiver.

Interventions Related to Wandering

Behavior: Exit-Seeking Wandering

Environmental Interventions

- Decrease the noise and confusion level.
- Eliminate the phone or overhead page (some units or facilities do this for 1–2 hours a day to create a "quiet time").
- Use simple signs and way-finding cues.
- Personalize residents' rooms.
- Put up "BioBoards." These are described in Table 10.3 and Figure 10.2.
- Set up multiple socializing and seating areas.
- Provide textures and objects to touch.
- Try childproof doorknob covers.

- Use "stop" signs.
- Develop enclosed outdoor and indoor wandering areas.
- Set up a "touch room" with many safe things in it.
- Make the environment more homelike—use aprons instead of bibs and incandescent lamps as well as fluorescent lights.
- Decrease through traffic if possible.
- Use personal wander bracelet alarms (Wanderguard, Secure Care).
- Develop a mobilizing system for alerting facility staff that a resident is missing—Code 10. A procedure for this is outlined in Table 10.4.
- Plan proactively with family, police, etc. for the possibility that a resident may wander away.
- Install coded doors.
- Disguise or camouflage doors. (Check with the local fire marshal to assure that this is acceptable. Some may discourage or prohibit this practice.)

Psychosocial/Activity Interventions

- Use distraction.
- Identify and follow the person's agenda.
- Go along with the resident—out one door and in another.
- Find ways to meet the resident's need to feel needed, secure, busy, and loved, by giving tasks and tools. (One woman, when given a cobbler apron, a feather duster, a dust rag, and a carpet sweeper, no longer wandered outside or into others' spaces.)
- Have the resident's family make a video- or audiotape and play it for the individual or try a collage of pictures.
- Use touch and hugs.
- Have reminiscence and picture boxes and bins available for staff, family, and volunteers to use with the resident (see chapter 14).

This is a suggested outline for a "Bioboard." Use dark pen and large print so it is easy to read.

Important People:

Resident:

Parents:

Brother(s) and sister(s):

Spouse: Spouses:

Children:

- - - - - - - - - - - - - - - - - -

Large picture of resident. Let resident if able, choose it.

- - - - - - - - - - - - - - - - - -

Grandchildren: Spouses:

Special/significant past or present events or hobbies

Greatgrandchildren: Spouses:

1.

2.

3.

4.

Other important people:

FIGURE 10.2   Bioboard outline.

- Take two to four residents at a time for walks, inside and outside the building.
- Take the resident with staff members who need to make short errands in the car.
- Personalize activities to fit with the resident's previous life experiences: if the resident sorted mail, give him a box of junk mail to sort.

Table 10.3   Instructions for Use of Bioboard

Several facilities have used Bioboards as a magician's tool to help a staff member "become" the resident. This piece of poster board containing information relevant to the resident (see Figure 10.2 for outline), such as a large picture of the resident (5" × 7") and a list and/or pictures of several significant events and people, is placed outside the door of the room. If the resident is cognitively and physically capable, he/she is consulted about whether or not he/she would like this done. If so, the resident can work with family or a volunteer to complete it. If the person is cognitively impaired, the family is encouraged to complete the Bioboard with the resident. For those with cognitive impairment, the events and pictures that will be most useful are from the past. It is important to keep information brief and write dark and large so that the information is easily visible. The purposes of the board include

- helping residents identify their rooms
- affirming for themselves and others who they were and are
- providing information to staff, family, and friends so that they can discuss relevant topics
- providing an opportunity for the family and resident to reflect on the life of the individual in all its fullness and meaning

Facilities have reported powerful results when biographical information is displayed in some way. One facility sends out a letter and outline to families in the admission packet. One of their severely disoriented and impaired residents, no longer able to recognize her family, had been in the Ice Follies in her youth. She drew staff and visitors to her door with a tremendous glow of pride, joy, and recognition after her picture with her ice skates was placed outside her door on the Bioboard.

Table 10.4 Mobilizing Staff to Find "Missing" Resident: (Code 10)

Procedure to carry out when patient/resident is missing from unit/facility.

Purpose: To find patient/resident as quickly as possible and maintain his/her safety, dignity, and privacy.

Missing patient/resident to be treated with same sense of immediacy as if it were a fire alarm.

Staff persons involved: All facility staff.

Nurse in charge of patient/resident directs search or consults with DNS, RN, or administrator.

Procedure: Inform the nurse in charge of patient/resident when discovered missing.

Nurse's responsibility:

1. Alert staff in building in the following way: using overhead page say: "Code 10. Will————[missing patient/resident name] please return to————[the unit]." Staff from other units call unit where patient is missing to get description if needed.
2. Staff on all units immediately look for patient/resident, making sure that all areas within building are searched.
3. On telephone, call unit from which patient is missing after area is thoroughly searched and report completed search.
4. After person is found, the nurse on the unit from which patient was missing uses overhead page and says, "Code 10 all clear."
5. Direct search to facility grounds if it is determined that patient/resident is not in building; remain in building and coordinate search (spend only a few minutes searching the grounds).
6. If patient/resident is not found immediately, call fire department or police and report that a patient/resident is missing.
7. When patient/resident is found and returned to center, examine for any possible injuries and treat accordingly.
8. Complete Incident Report if any injuries or if the person was missing for an extended period of time.
9. Record/report incident.

Behavior: Wandering into Others' Spaces or into Unsafe Spaces

Environmental Interventions

- Try a door guard, vinyl or Velcro barrier (guidelines for creating these are given in Table 10.5).
- Use Dutch doors (check to see if they meet the fire code).
- Use "stop" signs.
- Try dark tape strips, a grid, or a "black hole" on the floor in front of the doorway.
- Try exit alarms.

Psychosocial/Activity Interventions

- Use distraction.
- Anticipate and redirect the resident's actions.
- Identify any agenda the person has and try to meet it in another way.
- Provide companionship—family, volunteers, links with other residents, pets, or dolls.
- Have the resident attend activities on and off the unit.
- Determine the resident's past interests and activity patterns and provide similar activities when possible.

Interventions Related to Disruptive or Physically Aggressive Behavior

There is a high correlation between agitation and physical problems such as pain, illness, and medication side effects, so these need to be carefully assessed. General interventions that are effective for disruptive or aggressive behavior include the following:

- Provide a quiet, homelike environment.
- Work with staff to improve their verbal and nonverbal communication skills and techniques.

Table 10.5   Door Guards: Vinyl Door Barrier for Wanderers

The vinyl door barrier is a visual barrier that prevents wanderers from entering other residents' space or unsafe spaces, allowing mentally alert residents access without creating social isolation for either group.

Materials Needed

Bright yellow or other colored vinyl-coated nylon (Vicon 18) or other strong canvas type material 11 inches by 48 inches (the width of the resident's room door plus facings)

2 11-inch Velcro strips; get the kind with the self-stick soft strip to put on door frame and sew the hook side strip onto the vinyl. It is important to have the hook strip on the vinyl rather than the door jamb because the hooks on the Velcro will catch on clothes, etc., that brush against it.

Cut the vinyl to appropriate size and sew on the Velcro hook strip.

Peel off back of self-stick Velcro soft strip.

Place soft strip on door jamb at a height that seems appropriate. For many, 36 inches from the floor is good. Height will depend on whether the wanderer is a wheelchair or "foot" ambulator. If by wheelchair, you may wish to place it lower. About chest level seems to work best.

Advantages

- Low cost-materials cost about $7.50; often you can get a volunteer to sew it.
- It is aesthetically pleasing.
- It is easily cleaned.
- Velcro may be readily available in facility.
- It works really well for many residents.

Disadvantages: It takes time to arrange to have the barrier made; you have to find a volunteer and locate appropriate materials.

This idea was developed by Helen McGovern, RN; Delpha Duckett, RN; and Linda Learn, social worker, Mennonite Home in Albany, Oregon.

- Identify on care plans three things that provide comfort to residents when they become agitated, and also indicate what their anxious behaviors look, feel, and sound like before they escalate into a major episode so that staff can intercede early and prevent escalation.

- Try rocking chairs. They often are soothing for people who are agitated.
- Encourage the staff to allow and facilitate a sense of personalization and territoriality.
- Educate the staff about ways to prevent agitation and techniques to safely manage episodes of agitation.

Behavior: Biting

Environmental Interventions

- Place a towel over the staff member's shoulder to prevent biting during transfer.
- Have staff members wear heavy jackets during activities such as transfers.

Psychosocial/Activity Interventions

- Do not overwhelm the resident with many caregivers at once.
- Explain slowly what you are trying to do and move slowly, to prevent catastrophic reactions.
- Try giving the resident gum or candy to chew if it is safe.
- Provide textures and touch for stimulation.

Behavior: Pinching, Grabbing, Scratching

Environmental Interventions

- Give the person something soft to hold onto—a rolled up washrag, doll, or stuffed animal.
- Keep the resident's fingernails short.

Psychosocial/Activity Interventions

- Determine the cause of the grabbing (e.g., fear of falling or desire to keep someone with the person); try to meet the need calmly.
- Ask the person to "open your hand."

Behavior: Throwing

Environmental Interventions

- Provide soft foam balls to throw, and play catch with the resident.
- If utensils or plates are thrown at mealtimes, use finger foods.

Psychosocial/Activity Interventions

- Determine what meaning throwing may have for the resident (e.g., anger, part of a sport, or recreation).
- Play catch with a safe foam ball or beach ball.

Behavior: Hitting

Environmental Interventions

- Remove the person from high-activity areas.
- Try playing calming music with a tape recorder or personal headset.

Psychosocial/Activity Interventions

- Provide routine gentle touch and pleasing sensory stimulation and contact when the resident is calm, apart from care activities.
- Be sure staff members know how to prevent aggression and how to manage potentially dangerous situations.
- Use sudden distraction, like loud calling of the resident's name or clapping, when the person is about to strike out.
- Separate individuals who bring out negative behaviors in each other.
- Try one-to-one activities if the individual does poorly in a group.

Behavior: Kicking

Environmental Interventions

- Avoid approaching the resident from the front.

- Avoid kneeling in front of the resident; for example. If you know the resident may kick when his shoes are put on or off, do this with the resident in bed instead of sitting up.

Psychosocial/Activity Interventions

- Carefully observe and assess the resident's mood before approaching her.
- Use verbal and nonverbal skills to calm the resident.
- Try relaxation tapes, Walkman, or soothing music during care activities.

Behavior: Hair Pulling

Environmental Interventions

These interventions are the same as those for hitting and kicking.

Psychosocial/Activity Interventions

- Prevent the resident from pulling your hair by placing your hand over his to keep it close to the scalp.
- Maintain calm, friendly voice tones and facial expressions.
- Interventions to prevent hitting and kicking are also applicable here.

Behavior: Yelling

Be sure that the resident has been adequately evaluated or treated for pain. Yelling may be his only way to let you know of his discomfort.

Environmental Interventions

- Move the resident to a quieter place or decrease the noise in the environment.
- Change the resident's position.
- Consider removing or lowering the volume on the PA system and phone, or institute quiet hours with the PA off.

Psychosocial/Activity Interventions

- Ask the resident why he is yelling. (You get some interesting answers!)
- Provide touch and soothing verbal reassurance.
- Provide something warm and soft for the person to hug or hold.
- Try putting a Walkman stereo and earphones on the resident with some of his favorite music.

Behavior: Threatening (Verbal and Nonverbal)

Be sure you have adequately evaluated the resident for physical and medical problems such as pain and infections.

Environmental Interventions

- Try decreasing noxious stimuli by removing the resident from a high-activity area.
- Try increasing pleasurable stimuli by playing soothing or favorite music on a Walkman, or provide soft toys or massage.

Psychosocial/Activity Interventions

- Evaluate how staff activities and approaches affect behavior—is the resident responding defensively because he feels threatened?
- Determine the resident's past patterns of coping and interacting and the possible meaning of threats.
- Try one-to-one calming sensory stimulation activities such as back rubs or soft singing.
- Try distraction.
- Provide things to fiddle with, fold, or manipulate.

Behavior: Inappropriate Sexual Behaviors

These behaviors occur in persons with dementia for many reasons. If they are new or inconsistent with previous life patterns they may represent a loss of inhibitions, low self-esteem, or need for touch.

Finding the underlying meaning of the behavior and ruling out any physical problems and medication side effects is a critical first step.

Environmental Interventions

- Be aware that residents may misinterpret personal care activities that occur in "private spaces" like the bathroom or bedroom as sexual behavior.
- Provide privacy for residents who wish to masturbate unless they are causing self-harm.

Psychosocial/Activity Interventions

- When approaching a resident to do personal care activities, try addressing the resident formally, as "Mr. Smith" instead of "Sam," and clearly state that you are a nurse or CNA.
- Provide safe touching and contact in public areas such as the lounge by sitting across the table and holding hands.
- Try complimenting the person on his or her appearance to boost the sense of masculinity/femininity. Do this separately from personal care. Inappropriate sexual expression may occur because the person has unmet needs related to self-esteem.
- State clearly and firmly that the behavior is not appropriate or comfortable for you and ask the person to stop.
- Put on the resident's favorite cologne or aftershave to help improve his self-image.
- Provide hand, back, and foot rubs in a public place, not a private area.

Behavior: Self-mutilating (Pinching, Scratching, Hitting Self)

Be sure you have thoroughly investigated all possible physical causes or problems and the possible need for medical treatment.

Environmental Interventions

- Try using various types of gloves (garden, rubber, white, leather) and mitts or socks over the hand.

- Use air splints to prevent bending at the elbow only as a last resort after other interventions have failed.

Psychosocial/Activity Interventions

- Provide sensory stimulation and soothing touch.
- Provide positive sensory stimulation such as a sock massage by putting an angora sock over your hand and rubbing the extremities, face, etc., or use a blow dryer on a gentle, warm setting to blow air over the resident.
- Provide objects to hold, touch, or manipulate.

Behavior: Interference with Vital Treatment

Evaluate the benefit and burden of treatment from the resident's perspective. Caregivers and families often choose treatments for residents that they themselves would not wish to endure. The magician's work is crucial for seeing the treatment choice from the perspective of the resident's quality of life. Restrictive interventions should be implemented only as a last resort after this assessment.

Environmental Interventions

- Use an air splint to prevent bending at the elbow.
- Cover IV sites with a stockinette sleeve to keep them out of sight.
- Try gloves, mitts, socks over the resident's hand.

Psychosocial/Activity Interventions

- Arrange for family, staff, friends, or volunteers to sit with the person.
- Provide the person with something else to "fiddle" with, such as a towel tied in knots and anchored to the bed or wheelchair, a soft ball, or a piece of tubing.
- Allow the resident to explore the treatment equipment with supervision.

Other Interventions

- Continue working on regaining natural eating ability when possible.
- If the problem is an NG tube, consider the possibility of a gastric tube to lessen discomfort, and decrease accessibility of the tube.
- On IV or tube sites, try using different types of tape and/or as little tape as possible. Itchy tape often causes residents to pull on the site.
- Use a transparent dressing like as a base for tape rather than skin; it is not as irritating and eroding.

FALL PREVENTION AND MANAGEMENT

Maggie Donius

FALLS AND AGING

A variety of factors make older people more prone to falling. Normal aging changes as well as pathologies common in older people increase the risk of falling. Changes associated with aging that may increase the risk of falling include a shift in the center of gravity; flexion at the hips and knees; a stiffer, shuffling gait; decreased proprioception; decreased righting reflexes; increased response time; decreased ability to adjust to new environments; increased sensitivity to medications; and sensory deficits (hearing/vision).

Pathologies that are not a normal consequence of aging but are *common* in older people and increase the risk of falling include central nervous system disorders, dizziness or vertigo, drop attacks, orthostatic hypotension, syncope, and multiple chronic diseases. These disorders, if present, generally require medical intervention/management.

MANAGEMENT AND PREVENTION OF FALLS

While most falls, or unintentional changes in position, occur in persons over the age of 65, a majority of these falls do not result in serious injury. The literature indicates that, only 5%–15% of falls nationally result in serious injury. For example, in Oregon at one restraint-free facility providing care to physically and mentally frail elders, the percentage of falls that resulted in fractures has ranged from 1.5 to 2.3 for the past 4 years. Yet we often intervene as if all falls caused serious injury.

Erring on the side of overprotection and restricting mobility creates a new set of problems. The complications of immobility can be deadly, especially for the frail elderly. After a fall, fear of falling itself can drastically limit mobility. Therefore, it is critical that care providers assess the risks and causes of falls. Performing a mobility/fall risk assessment and sharing the outcome with the resident, the family, and the staff is important. It is also essential to seek agreement from the resident, family, and staff on an acceptable margin of safety and formulate interventions to provide or improve that margin of safety. These interventions should be communicated to all involved and the risks and benefits of the interventions assessed on an ongoing basis.

A key strategy in fall prevention is to decrease the number of risk factors and, whenever possible, maximize the person's abilities. Areas to explore include acute and chronic illnesses, medications, environmental hazards, and sensory function.

Educating the involved parties about aging changes that increase the risk of falling, existing medical conditions or health problems that may contribute to this risk, and the individual's ability or lack of ability is critical in establishing realistic expectations for fall prevention. It is important for residents, family, and staff to understand that no magical protection comes with being in a health care institution.

Management of Acute and Chronic Illnesses

It is important to make sure that chronic illnesses such as diabetes, congestive heart failure (CHF), hypertension, and so on are well controlled. It is equally important to recognize and treat acute illnesses such as urinary tract and respiratory tract infections. Adequate and appropriate treatment of acute and chronic illnesses requires recognition of atypical presentations of illness, which may include change in mental and/or functional status, or falls.

When looking for possible causes of falls, it may be helpful to obtain
1. lab work, such as
   a. CBC
   b. Na, K, Ca, glucose, creatinine, etc.
   c. thyroid function test
   d. Urinalysis (UA) if possibly symptomatic
2. ECG or Holter monitoring if cardiac problems are *highly* suspected as the cause of falls.

If abnormalities are found and corrected, fall risk will decrease if these abnormalities were contributing to the falls.

MEDICATIONS

Certain medications or combinations of medications can increase one's risk or tendency to fall. Consulting a pharmacist can be extremely helpful when considering medications as a potential cause of falls. Medications thought to be particularly problematic include analgesics, diuretics, hypnotics, nonsteroidal antiinflammatory drugs, antipsychotics, and tricyclic antidepressants.

ENVIRONMENT

Hazards in the environment can also cause or contribute to falls. It is helpful to create an environment that considers aging changes and is as free of hazards as possible. Lighting may be too dim or may contribute to glare and/or create shadows. Walking surfaces that are uneven, slippery, or patterned may contribute to falls. Step edges that are not clearly defined can pose particular risks. Furniture that is too low or too soft, tips easily, or is on wheels can also create problems. Slippery tubs or showers, as well as lack of grab rails for tub and toilet, can make bathrooms hazardous. Shoes and slippers that are too loose, badly worn, or have slick soles can contribute to falls. Clothing that is too long, loose, or flowing can also cause problems. Broken or improperly used equipment is also hazardous (Stone & Chenitz, 1991). Although restraints and siderails were once thought to be safety devices, the literature indicates that they often increase the injury sustained in a fall. Further, individuals who are restrained may lose the ability to ambulate in as short a time as 2–3 weeks. Restraints have been the cause or contributed to death in many cases (Miles & Irvine, 1992).

The "You see it, you own it, you deal with it now" attitude must prevail when environmental hazards such as liquid on the floor are noticed. These hazards must be dealt with immediately. Nightlights and a clear pathway can facilitate safe trips to the toilet. Shiny floors have long been mentioned as a possible causative factor in falls. Aging changes in the eye make the glare from highly polished floors problematic. Stripping away wax and using sealer instead, along with low rather than high buffing, is one method of protecting the floor without producing high gloss. Antiskid acrylic wax is another alternative.

Sensory Function

Facilitating and enhancing sensory function is an important part of fall prevention so that cues from the environment can be maximized. In particular, a vision screening test should be done in the facility and the resident referred for treatment if problems are suspected or found. If they are needed, glasses should be worn, and they should be clean and the prescription up to date. Ears that are occluded with wax should be evaluated for cleansing. Hearing aids, if used, should be in and working (most batteries last about $1\frac{1}{2}$ to 2 weeks if taken out at night).

Mobility and Fall Risk Assessment

Assessing mobility and fall risk is a key step in a fall prevention/management plan. Several tools can be used to perform a systematic assessment. These include the Get Up and Go Go Test, the Morse Fall Scale, and the Tinetti Balance and Gait Evaluation.

The Get Up and Go Go Test is a variation of the "get up and go" test developed by Mathias, Nayak, and Isaacs (1986). The second "Go" represents the addition of toileting observation. This was added because of the high frequency of falls that occur during attempts to go to and from the bathroom.

To do the Get Up and Go Go test, observe the person

a. sit and stand from a chair
b. turn around (360°) while standing
c. walk or wheel to the bathroom or toilet
d. get onto and use the toilet, including clothing management, etc.
e. get off the toilet and get into wheelchair if used
f. walk or wheel from the toilet/bathroom to the bed
g. get into and out of bed

Following observation of the person doing the Get Up and Go Go Test, document his ability to perform *a–g* above. Decisions about the safety of independent transfer, trips to the bathroom, and so on can be based on the outcome of this assessment. The assessment is brief, so it can be repeated as many times as necessary. This is especially important if the older person's ability varies over the course of the day.

Documentation of the observation of this test might look like this.

Example 1

- Subjective data: At home I got up at night on my own to use the toilet.
- Objective data: Able to sit and stand from room chair by pushing up with arms on arms of chair on first attempt. Turned 360 degrees slowly, without loss of balance. Walked to and from bathroom, used toilet, including clothing management, and got into and out of bed independently without difficulty.
- Assessment: Safe in independent ambulation, transfer, and toilet use at this time.
- Plan: Talk with resident, his wife and staff about leaving siderails down to facilitate independent bathroom use.

Example 2

- Subjective data: I have to use the toilet several times during the night. I've tried not drinking fluids after dinner, but I still have to go.
- Objective data: Able to sit and stand from chair brought from home by pushing with arms on arms of chair, but several attempts required to stand. Turns 360 degrees while standing by repositioning feet and walker 9 times. Stood for several seconds before ambulating. Walked to and from bathroom with wheeled walker. Unable to manage clothing as did not let go of walker until seated. Used grab bar to rise from toilet and walked with walker to bed. Able to get into bed but unable to come from supine to sitting position even when pulling on siderail.
- Assessment: Mobility deficits do not allow independent supine to sitting and clothing management for toilet use.
- Plan: Discuss with resident using the call light to summon help during the night or independent use of the bed pan if able, and use of call light to have pan emptied. Explore physical and or occupational therapy consultation. Ask for her ideas and implement if possible. Document resident's decision on plan of care.

Documenting in this way links the resident's ability to the rationale and the plan/intervention.

Balance and Gait Evaluation

When it is apparent that mobility problems are present, the 16-item Tinetti Balance and Gait Evaluation (shown in Table 11.1) can be helpful (Tinetti, 1986; Tinetti, Williams, & Mayewski, 1986). The resident is observed performing the activities listed on the tool and is scored as indicated on the form. The score is the number of points the resident earns; the maximum possible on the balance portion of the tool is 16, and the maximum possible on gait is 12, or 28 total points possible. Problems can then be pinpointed and interventions targeted. The results can be used to demonstrate need for physical therapy intervention and perhaps document improvement.

Fall Risk Assessment

The Morse Fall Scale (shown in Table 11.2) is a 6-item scale that assesses fall risk and can be used as a guide to interventions. It is quick and easy to administer. The instrument has been tested in long-term care, rehabilitation, and acute care. There is no medication item on the scale—not an omission; it is felt that medication effects show up in gait. The score can be used to help make decisions about who is at high risk of falling and can assist in targeting interventions. Each facility needs to decide on a cutoff score for high risk.

If a fall risk assessment (like the Morse Fall Scale) is not done routinely at the time of admission, it is important to determine if an older person has a history of falling. Those who fall—"fallers"— tend to fall again. Section K (Health Conditions) of the MDS (Minimum Data Set), an assessment tool required by federal regulations on all nursing home residents, addresses this issue for a 180-day period, but it may not be completed until 14 days after admission. This may be too late. Asking family members and/or previous caregivers about falls is important because falls that do not result in serious injury are often not remembered or reported.

STRATEGIES TO INCREASE SAFETY

Gathering Information on Falls

Collecting and analyzing information about falls, which is generally present on incident reports, is an important component of a fall prevention/management program. A fall and subsequent incident report do not mean that someone did not do his job. Incident reports provide clues in an investigation; they are not fault-finding or blame-placing tools unless this is warranted. This is especially true when people are suffering from dementia and cannot provide

Table 11.1 Tinetti Balance and Gait Evaluation

BALANCE

Instructions: The subject begins this assessment seated in a backless (or straight-backed), armless, firm chair. A *walking aid* is defined as a cane or walker. Circle the appropriate score.

1. *Sitting balance*
Leans or slides down in chair	= 0
Steady, stable, safe	= 1

2. *Rising from chair*
Unable without human assistance	= 0
Able but uses arms (on chair or walking aid) to pull or push up	= 1
Able to rise in a single movement without using arms on chair or walking aid (Note: use of arms on subject's own thighs scores a 2)	= 2

3. *Attempts to rise*
Unable without human assistance	= 0
Able but requires multiple attempts	= 1
Able to rise with one attempt	= 2

4. *Immediate standing balance (first 3–5 seconds)*
Any sign of unsteadiness (defined as grabbing at object for support, staggering, moving feet, or more than minimal trunk sway)	= 0
Steady but USES WALKING AID or grabs other object for support	= 1
Steady without holding onto walking aid or other object for support	= 2

5. *Standing balance*
Any sign of unsteadiness regardless of stance, or holds onto object	= 0
Steady but *wide stance* (defined as medial heels more than 40″ apart) or USES WALKING AID or other support	= 1
Steady *narrow stance* (defined as medial heels less than 40″ apart) and without holding onto any object for support	= 2

(continued)

Table 11.1 *Continued*

6. *Nudge on sternum* (with subject standing with feet as close together as possible, examiner pushes with light even pressure over sternum three times; reflects ability to withstand displacement)

Begins to fall or examiner has to help maintain balance	= 0
Needs to move feet but able to maintain balance (e.g., staggers, grabs, but catches self)	= 1
Steady, able to withstand pressure	= 2

7. *Balance with eyes closed* (with subject standing with feet as close together as possible with arms at sides, examiner counts out 5 seconds)

Any sign of unsteadiness or needs to hold onto an object	= 0
Steady without holding onto any object with feet close together	= 1

8. *Turning balance* (360°) (from a standing still position, have the subject turn around in a 360° circle, demonstrate this first and give the subject one chance to practice)   = 0

Steps are *discontinuous* (define as subject puts one foot completely on the floor before raising the other foot)	= 1
Steps are *continuous* (defined as the turn is a flowing movement)	= 1
Any sign of unsteadiness or holds onto an object	= 0
Steady without holding onto any object	= 1

9. *Sitting down*

Unsafe (falls into chair, misjudges distances, lands off-center)	= 0
Needs to use arms to guide self into chair or not a smooth movement	= 1
Able to sit down in one safe, smooth motion	= 2

Balance Score: /16

GAIT

Instructions: The subject stands with the examiner. They walk down the hallway or across a room (preferably where there are few people or obstacles). The subject should be told to walk at his/her "usual" pace using his/her usual walking aid. Circle the appropriate score.

(continued)

Table 11.1 *Continued*

10. *Initiation of gait* (subject is asked to begin walking down
    the hallway immediately after being told to "go")
    Any hesitancy, multiple attempts to start, or initiation of   = 0
    gait not a smooth motion
    Subject begins walking immediately without observable   = 1
    hesitation and initiation of gait is a single, smooth motion

11. *Step length and height* (Observe distance between toe of
    stance foot and heel of swing foot, observe from the side,
    do not judge first few steps, observe one foot at a time)
    Right swing foot does *not pass* left stance foot with each   = 0
    step
    Right swing foot *passes* left stance foot with each step   = 1
    Right swing foot does not clear floor completely with each   = 0
    step (may hear scraping) or is raised markedly high
    (e.g., due to drop foot)
    Right swing foot completely clears floor but is not   = 1
    markedly high
    Left swing foot does *not pass* right stance foot with each   = 0
    step
    Left swing foot *passes* right stance foot with each step   = 1
    Left foot does *not clear* floor completely with each step   = 0
    (may hear scraping) or is raised markedly high (e.g., due
    to drop foot)
    Left swing foot completely clears floor but is not markedly   = 1
    high

12. *Step Symmetry* (observed distance between toe of each
    stance foot and heel of each swing foot, observe from the
    side, do not judge first few steps)
    Step length varies between sides or resident advances with   = 0
    same foot with every step
    Step length same or nearly same on both sides for most   = 1
    step cycles

13. Steps are *discontinuous* (defined as subject places entire   = 0
    foot, heel and toe, on floor before beginning to raise
    other foot) or subject stops completely between steps

(continued)

Table 11.1 *Continued*

Steps are *continuous* (defined as subject begins raising heel of one foot as heel of other foot touches the floor) and there are no breaks or stops in subject's stride	= 1

14. *Path deviation* (observe in relation to floor tiles or a line on the floor, observe one foot over several strides—about 10 ft of path length, observe from behind; difficult to assess if subject uses a walking aid)

    Marked deviation of foot from side-to-side or toward one direction   = 0

    Mild/moderate deviation, or subject USES A WALKING AID   = 1

    Foot follows close to a straight line as subject advances   = 2

15. *Trunk stability* (observe from behind)

    Marked side-to-side trunk sway or subject USES A WALKING AID   = 0

    No side-to-side trunk sway, but subject flexes knees or back or subject spreads arms out while walking   = 1

    Trunk does not sway, knees and back are not flexed, arms are not abducted in an effort to maintain stability   = 2

16. *Walk stance* (observe from behind)

    Feet apart with stepping   = 0

    Feet should almost touch as one foot passes the other   = 1

Gait score: /12
Total score: /28

From Tiretti, M., (1986), Performance-oriented assessment of mobility problems in elderly patients *Journal of the American Genatries Society*, 34(2), 119–126. Reprinted with permission.

information about the circumstances of their fall. Asking those who complete the incident report (those most familiar with the fall) to list something that could be done to prevent a recurrence of the fall can stimulate ideas for intervention and prevention. This adds a new focus—prevention—to what has traditionally been only a report of events. The faller should be asked to describe the circumstances of the fall if he is able, for this can provide important clues about the cause and perhaps prevent future falls.

The fall tracking form (see Figure 11.1) lists the date, time, and

Table 11.2   Morse Fall Scale

1. History of falling	no	0	_____
	yes	25	_____
2. Secondary diagnosis	no	0	_____
	yes	15	_____
3. Ambulatory aid			
none/bedrest/nurse assist		0	_____
crutches/cane/walker		15	_____
furniture		30	_____
4. Intravenous therapy/heparin lock	no	0	_____
	yes	20	_____
5. Gait			
normal/bedrest/wheelchair		0	_____
weak		10	_____
impaired		20	_____
6. Mental status			
oriented to own ability		0	_____
overestimates/forgets limitations		15	_____

Total _____

Definition of Variables for the Morse Fall Scale

History of falling
> Yes (scored 25) if a previous fall is recorded during the present admission or if there is immediate history of physiological falls (i.e., from seizures, impaired gait) prior to admission.

Secondary diagnosis
> Yes (15) if more than one medical diagnosis is listed on the patient chart.

Ambulatory aids
> Scored 0 if patient walks without a walking aid even if assisted by a nurse or is on bedrest.
> Scored 15 if ambulatory with crutches, cane, or walker.
> Scored 20 if clutches onto furniture for support.

Intravenous therapy
> Scored 20 if has an IV apparatus or heparin lock.

Gait
> Normal gait scored 0 if patient is able to walk with head erect, arms swinging freely at the side, and strides unhesitantly.

(continued)

Table 11.2 *Continued*

Weak gait scored 10 if patient is stooped but able to lift head while walking. Furniture support may be sought but is of feather-weight touch, almost for reassurance. Steps are short, and the patient may shuffle.

Impaired gait scored 20 if patient is stooped, may have difficulty rising from the chair, attempts to rise by pushing on the arms of the chair and/or by "bouncing." The patient's head is down, and because balance is poor the patient grasps the furniture, a person, or walking aid for support and cannot walk without assistance. Steps are short and patient shuffles.

If patient is wheelchair-bound, the patient is scored according to the gait s/he uses when transferring from the wheelchair to the bed.

Mental Status

The patient is asked if s/he is able to go to the bathroom alone or if s/he needs assistance or if s/he is permitted up. If the patient's response is consistent with the ambulatory orders on the Kardex, the score is 0.

If the response is not consistent with the orders or if the patient's assessment is unrealistic, score is 15.

The authors suggest each institution determine its own cutoff for high risk.

Morse, J. M., Morse, R. M., & Tylko, S. J. (1989). Development of a scale to identify the fall-prone patient. *Canadian Journal on Aging*, 8(4), 366–377. Reprinted with permission.

activity underway at the time of the fall. This is a useful tool because it can reveal patterns or trends in a particular resident's falls. Incident reports that contain this and other information are not readily available after completion. Thus, information that might provide clues to the cause and perhaps prevention of falls, especially if the resident is cognitively impaired, is locked away in a file cabinet. The staff may not be aware of falls that take place on another shift or on their days off. Getting information about previous falls to the staff and other care providers, so that it can be used for the benefit of the faller, is critical. The fall tracking form should be placed so that those providing direct care to the resident can see the number, time, and circumstances of falls. The fall tracking form can be used as a investigative worksheet/tool as well as an alerting device for staff. Facility administration may want to decide if the information should become part of the resident's record or if it is to be used simply as a data-gathering tool to help develop interventions.

Falls occur for many reasons. After evaluating the information recorded on the fall tracking form, care providers can often make an educated guess about probable causes of falls and develop specific strategies to decrease the risk. These strategies may include the following:

- Falls occurring before meals may be caused by low blood sugar. Snacks and/or medication adjustment may prevent these falls.

- Falls after meals may be caused by postprandial hypotension. Staying seated or being accompanied after meals may prevent these falls.

- Falls that occur with standing or transfer may be due to orthostatic hypotension. Drug review, medical evaluation and intervention are necessary.

- Falls that occur with head movement (looking side to side or up) may be caused by carotid or vertebral artery compression that impairs circulation to the brain. Medical evaluation should be sought.

- If elimination is frequently involved (i.e., falls occur in or on the way to the bathroom, there is urine on the floor, etc.), systematically addressing toileting needs may prevent further falls.

- Falls might be medication-related (after pain medication, on the days when a diuretic is given); a pharmacy consult may be helpful.

- Falls that tend to occur later in the day may be caused by fatigue. A scheduled nap or down time may prevent or decrease these falls.

- Falls can be a sign of an acute illness (UTI, respiratory infection) or a flare up of a chronic disease (diabetes, CHF, etc.) that has not been detected or treated. Assessment and treatment of these problems are indicated.

Use this information to detect patterns of falls and their possible cause.

Date	Time	Activity at time of fall	Other

Name: _____

D0156.12

FIGURE 11.1 Fall tracking form.

If the information on the fall tracking form reveals no pattern or trend (i.e., the falls tend to occur haphazardly or for "no reason at all"), intervention may not be possible other than keeping the environment as safe as possible, maximizing the resident's abilities, and crossing your fingers. Sharing this conclusion with residents who are able to understand and with families and staff is important. They can cross their fingers too.

In acute care settings, where length of stay is generally short, using some kind of sticker identification on the door and/or Kardex to alert staff to high-fall-risk patients has been reported to be effective. Although research to substantiate the efficacy of this intervention in long-term care is lacking, it may be helpful in communicating fall risk to staff. Completing and placing the fall tracking form, with fall risk information, in an appropriate location on the plan of care and CNA assignment sheet and communicating concerns about falls in the report are other strategies to increase staff awareness.

Education

It is important to educate the older person, the family, and staff about the causes of falls. All parties should have *realistic* expectations about fall prevention. A fall in a care institution does not automatically mean that someone did not do his job. An acceptable margin of safety should be agreed upon by all involved: the older person, family, staff, and, in some cases, the care institution. The benefits and burden of facilitating or restricting mobility should be considered when deciding on an acceptable margin of safety. Residents, families, and staff need to know that unless the cause of falls can be determined, prevention may not be possible. Interventions may need to focus on decreasing the injury rather than preventing the fall. The risks and benefits of allowing and facilitating freedom are the major issues to consider in negotiating a mutually agreeable margin of safety.

Litigation, especially when a fall results in serious injury, is a common fear. This fear may be a major causative factor in the safety-at-all-costs attitude. However, there has been more successful litigation in cases of use and misuse of restraints than for nonuse of restraints, although litigation can occur in either situation (Kapp, 1991). Now that research evidence demonstrates that physical restraints may do more harm than good, restraint use does not provide protection from litigation.

To avoid litigation, make decisions based on good assessments that have been shared with the people most likely to sue. Document the discussion and agreement about the acceptable margin of safety with those same individuals. It is important to make clear to those most likely to sue that there is no guarantee that falls will not occur. Explain that aid will be rendered immediately and that the necessary actions to ensure comfort and evaluation will be taken. Documenting the thoughtful process that has been carried out is important. Making sure that there is no conflict between the physician's order, staff actions, and the documented plan of care can also prevent litigation.

Dealing with Environmental Hazards

The fall tracking form information can indicate patterns of environmental hazards if they are present. Sometimes items that we consider safety devices may actually function as barriers to mobility and increase risk; these should not be used. Although the use of siderails is standard in many institutions, their efficacy in fall prevention has not been demonstrated (Rubenstein, Miller, Postel, & Evans, 1983). Climbing out of bed over siderails merely increases the height from which one might fall. Other potential negative consequences of siderails include separating the care receiver from the caregiver, serving as a potential trauma-causing agent, creating a guillotine-like noise when being raised and lowered, creating a sense of being jailed or trapped, obstructing vision, and accidentally dislodging tubes such as catheters. The decision to use or not use siderails should be based on a resident's wishes and the resident's ability to get into and out of bed safely. Residents who can respond should be asked if they want their siderails up or down. If they want them up, the reason should be documented, and it should be noted that it is the resident's choice. Residents who want their rails down and residents who cannot express their desire should be assessed. The behavior of residents who are unable to respond verbally should be considered. Residents who attempt to climb over the rails are usually indicating that the rails are a barrier to their mobility. It is generally appropriate to include family members in discussions about siderail use, but the desire of residents, when their desire can be determined, should always be given first consideration. When resident desires cannot be determined, the family and staff should come to a mutually agreeable plan based on the outcome of the assessment.

Siderail Assessment

A siderail assessment should include observation of the person getting into and out of bed unassisted with the rails down. For those who travel in a wheelchair, ability to get into and out of bed from and to that chair should be observed. Potential safety problems, such as not locking brakes, can then be detected in a systematic way. The assessment should be documented.

Siderail Assessment Example

Documentation of the assessment might look like this:

- Subjective: I don't want to wait. Sometimes they don't come when I call, and I don't want to wet the bed.
- Subjective: Staff report that wheelchair brakes have been explained multiple times but not remembered by resident.
- Objective: Approached bedside in wheelchair, stood without locking brakes, got into bed supporting self on bedside stand. Got to supine without difficulty, unable to come from supine to sitting. Raising the siderail on the wall side for support facilitated this position change. Was unable to retrieve the wheelchair, which rolled away during transfer to bed. When asked about the brakes, resident was unaware.
- Assessment: Safety of independent transfer is questionable due to not locking brakes of wheelchair, but resident may be able to use a stationary commode next to bed. Elevating siderail on wall side of bed facilitates supine to sitting position change.

- Plan: Assess resident's ability to safely use commode at bed-side with outside siderail down and siderail on wall side of bed up. Discuss with resident, family, and staff.

Categorizing Risk (Levels 1, 2, and 3)

When considering siderail use, residents generally can be catego-rized into three groups: those who are able to get into and out of bed safely, those who are unable to get into and out of bed safely or whose safety is questionable, and those who lack the ability to get into or out of bed.

Those who are able to get into and out of bed safely are at low risk (Level 1), so siderails are not necessary. This should be dis-cussed with the resident, family, and staff. When rails have been up, it may be wise to lower the rails gradually, starting during the day and working up to all the time so that continued assessment can be done.

If residents have the desire and attempt to get into and out of bed unassisted, one must consider whether they have demonstrated questionable safety during the assessment. If residents demon-strate questionable safety but have the desire or attempt to get into and out of bed unassisted, siderails or alternatives will be needed as they are at moderate or high risk (Level 2 or 3).

If they do not have the desire or do not initiate position changes, they are probably at low risk (Level 1) and do not need siderails or alternatives. This should be validated with the resident, family, and staff. Residents who are physically incapable of getting out of bed, for example, residents who move very little or are in a persistent vegetative state, are at low risk, and siderails serve little purpose. Siderails are usually up simply as a matter of policy or because they have always been up. The potential negative consequences of siderail use are seldom considered in these situations.

Are Siderails Restraints?

If it is determined through an assessment and through consultation with the resident, family, and staff that the resident would benefit from siderails, a determination needs to be made as to whether the rails are or are not a restraint. Siderails are considered to be restraints if their intended purpose is to restrict freedom of movement, such as preventing a resident from getting into or out of bed when he or she wishes. When siderails are used to restrict a resident's freedom of movement, a physician's order is needed, and the documentation generally required for restraint use is necessary. Usually, these are situations in which there are no alternatives, alternatives have failed, or the benefit of using siderails outweighs their burden. (See chapter 10 for a discussion of evaluating the benefits and burdens of restraints.)

Residents who do not have the desire or ability to leave the bed may have their rails up, but they are not considered restraints because freedom of movement is not being restricted. Rails in these cases are generally not necessary, as the risk is low; however, if the resident's desire cannot be determined and the family wants siderails up, the rails are not restraints. Siderails are also not restraints when the resident chooses to use them. The siderail decision tree (in Figure 11.2) illustrates the siderail assessment and decision-making process and gives specifics that may be helpful when considering and assessing siderail use.

Siderail elimination is not the goal. The goal is to individualize siderail use and use rails only when they truly increase the safety, security, and mobility of the residents in our care.

Other Care Approaches

Because older people have decreased warning time before urination, instructing them to wait for assistance may be unrealistic, especially for those with memory impairment and those not accustomed to needing or waiting for help. Placing a commode next to the bed if the person can safely use it is a continence-facilitating, safer option. Assess the safety of this intervention by observing the person getting out of bed, using the commode, and getting back into bed. Document this assessment as you would the Get Up and Go Go test. Discuss the results of the assessment with the resident, family, and staff to see if this is within an acceptable margin of safety. A nonslip, cleanable rug at the bedside will prevent slipping in urine if this is likely to occur. When cognitive impairment is present, facilitating or making safer what a resident is likely to do,

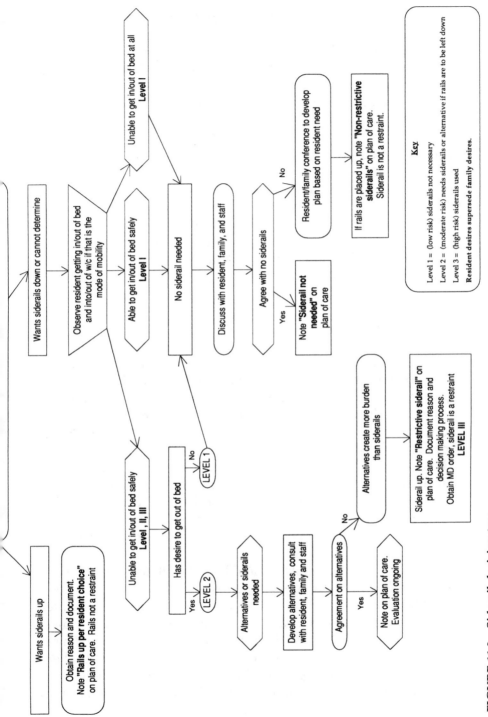

FIGURE 11.2 Siderail decision tree.

rather than attempting to make the resident stop the behavior, is often a wiser, safer, more realistic intervention. People suffering from dementia will generally not remember to use the call light even with frequent reminders, so we should not plan for them to do so.

Ongoing Assessment

Because residents, environment, and staffs change, it is important that the risks and benefits of fall prevention or management strategies be periodically reviewed. An immediate review (and documentation of that review) should occur with any change in the resident's condition. A notation should be made in the quarterly review even if the resident is stable and no changes are needed.

SUMMARY

Enhancing the abilities of older people and decreasing risk factors when possible are important components of preventing and managing falls. Assessing mobility and fall risk so that interventions can be individualized is critical. Detecting a pattern if one exists can pinpoint the cause as well as indicate appropriate corrective action for fall prevention.

It is vital to intervene when intervention has a possible positive outcome and to seek the agreement of all those involved. However, sometimes the "cure is worse than the disease." We must have the courage to seek agreement on not intervening when the burden of intervention outweighs the risk or the possible consequences of a fall.

The goal of care providers should be to facilitate the mobility of older people within an agreed-upon acceptable margin of safety, rather than hinder it or maintain safety at all costs. Shortly after mobility is restricted, the ability to be mobile is lost. The consequences of immobility can be just as devastating as the consequences of falls. The worst outcome in both cases is death. There are risks involved in helping frail older people to be mobile. Perhaps one of the most difficult tasks of health care professionals is to assist older people, their significant others, and society at large to accept and deal with these risks.

REFERENCES

Kapp, M. (1991). Reduce legal risks through restraint reduction plan. *Provider, 17*(8), 48–49.

Mathias, S., Nayak, U.S., & Isaacs, B. (1986). Balance in the elderly patient: The "get-up and go" test. *Archives of Physical Medicine and Rehabilitation, 67*(6), 387–389.

Miles, S.H., & Irvine, P. (1992). Deaths caused by physical restraints. *Gerontologist, 32*(6), 762–766.

Morse, J.M. (1986). Computerized evaluation of a scale to identify the fall-prone patient. *Canadian Journal of Public Health, 77*(1), 21–25.

Morse, J.M., Black, C., Oberle, K., & Donahue, P. (1989). A prospective study to identify the fall-prone patient. *Social Science and Medicine, 28*(1), 81–86.

Morse, J.M., Morse, R.M., & Tylko, S.J. (1989). Development of a scale to identify the fall-prone patient. *Canadian Journal on Aging, 8*(4), 366–377.

Morse, J.M., Tylko, S.J., & Dixon, H.A. (1987). Characteristics of the fall-prone patient. *Gerontologist, 27*(4), 516–522.

Rubenstein, H.S., Miller, F.H., Postel, S.F., & Evans, H.B. (1983). Standards of medical care based on consensus rather than evidence: The case of routine bedrail use for the elderly. *Law, Medicine & Health Care, 11*(6), 271–276.

Stone, J.K., & Chenitz, W.C. (1991). The problem of falls. In W.C. Chenitz, J.T. Stone, & S.A. Salisbury, (Eds.), *Clinical Gerontological Nursing. A Guide to Advanced Practice* (p. 300). Philadelphia: W.B. Saunders.

Tinetti, M. (1986). Performance-oriented assessment of mobility problems in elderly patients. *Journal of American Geriatric Society, 34*(2), 119–126.

Tinetti, M., Williams, T.F., & Mayewski, R. (1986). Fall risk index for elderly patients based on number of chronic disabilities. *American Journal of Medicine, 80*, 429–434.

A 12-minute video, "Using the More Fall Scale," is available for a fee, (Oct. 1994) from: Audiovisual Department, Glenrose Rehabilitation Hospital, 10230-111 Avenue, Edmonton, Alta. T5G 0B7, Canada (403)471-2262.

Chapter **12**

SEATING PROBLEMS IN LONG-TERM CARE

Deborah A. Jones

Most nursing home facilities are expected to provide wheelchairs for their residents. Traditionally, nursing homes have used wheelchairs that have sling seats and sling backs with fixed armrests and fixed leg rests. These chairs were designed for transport—for someone to push rather than for the occupant to wheel. They were not designed for long-term sitting needs. Still, they are the wheelchair most commonly found in nursing homes throughout the United States today, and residents are sitting in them for extended periods of time.

Several studies have found that as many as 80% of nursing home residents experience problems with their wheelchairs. A third of these problems are moderate to severe and include discomfort, inhibited mobility, and poor posture (Shaw & Taylor, 1992). The most common observation—and subsequent rationale for restraint use—is that the resident appears to be "sliding out of the wheelchair." Why?

Recent studies indicate that comfort is the top priority for residents in nursing homes; they want to be comfortable more than anything else. Unfortunately, sitting in a chair with a sling seat over a long period may not only be uncomfortable but may lead to a number of biomechanical problems. Hammocking leads to pelvic obliquity and poor lower extremity positioning.

Inadequate pelvic support and poor femoral loading results in kyphotic posture and resultant migration. Other problems can include sacral sitting and/or unsupported thighs that roll inward. Mechanical problems that can affect wheelchair safety and function include general disrepair, poor wheelchair alignment, and faulty wheel locks. A poorly fitted wheelchair includes wrong seat width and seat depth, inadequate foot support, and improper armrest height.

Although 70%–75% of nursing home residents are women, a majority of wheelchairs in the facilities are made for a person who is 6 feet tall and 18 inches wide. As a result, many residents are forced to sit in wheelchairs much too large for their stature. Their feet may not reach the ground or the footrests, causing increased pressure under their thighs. This may lead to circulatory problems and edema in their legs. To gain support under their feet, they typically scoot out to the edge of the chair to reach the floor. Once the hips have been displaced forward in the wheelchair, the lower back is left unsupported and the trunk collapses forward. This results in increased pressure across the upper back and can lead to skin breakdown and pain. Also, if this person tries to reach over the armrests while in this position, the axillary region may experience an increase in pressure from improper armrest height, resulting in neurologic and circulatory problems. In addition, upper extremity function is compromised when the trunk is poorly positioned. For instance, the arms feel heavier, which makes it more difficult to do small tasks such as raising the arms for eating or grooming, thumbing through magazines or playing cards, let alone propelling the wheelchair.

Poorly fitted seating may lead to compensations in posture, causing long-term compression of the trunk, which in turn may cause problems with circulation, gastrointestinal and urinary tract dysfunction, and high blood pressure. Poor seating may also lead to problems with speech, swallowing, chewing, and breathing. The resident may be unable to deliver a productive cough and achieve efficient lower lobe breathing, placing him or her at risk for pneumonia. Vital capacity may be compromised, requiring the heart to work harder, possibly leading to cardiac failure.

Inactivity caused by poor posture further compounds these risks. With proper positioning of the pelvis and trunk, a level eye gaze can be achieved, which increases the opportunity for improved communication and socialization. A resident who is seated properly can achieve more socialization and greater self-esteem and therefore a higher quality of life.

Allowing residents to function at their optimal level through appropriate seating and positioning will also result in less need for nursing and medical care.

Most seating problems can be easily corrected. Figure 12.1 illustrates a simple form that staff can use as part of the assessment of seating and mobility needs. After it is filled out, it can be shared with the physical therapist. The results are well worth the time it takes for observation, evaluation, simulation, recommendations, and application of equipment. For instance, a more comfortable resident will stay up in the wheelchair longer, with less pain or agitation. A resident who can self-propel his wheelchair will have the autonomy to go where he wishes. A resident who can pull the wheelchair up to the sink and see in the mirror can participate in self-care tasks such as grooming and hygiene. A resident who can talk with a loud voice, breathe freely, and swallow effectively will have more energy, greater endurance, and less chance of aspiration.

This chapter describes the functional goals for seating and positioning, the most common problems seen in long-term care, and some solutions to the problems. It concludes with a brief discussion of wheelchair equipment appropriate for long-term care residents.

FUNCTIONAL GOALS FOR SEATING

Goal 1: Independent Mobility

When residents are placed in a good position, with the correct wheelchair and seating, they have the potential to achieve a higher level of function. It is important to enable residents to move in the most efficient way. Some will use both legs, others both arms, and still others, a combination of arms and legs. Positioning with proper equipment should optimize the chosen method of wheelchair mobility.

Patient name:								Date:
Walking	Yes ☐ No ☐	W/Assist. ☐		Cane ☐		Walker ☐		Brace ☐
Wheelchair:	Yes ☐ No ☐	Uses arms ☐		Legs ☐		Electric ☐		
Sitting positioning:	Slouched ☐ Forward head ☐ Legs roll in ☐		Leans forward ☐ Legs too high ☐ Legs roll out ☐			Leans to one side ☐ Legs to low ☐ Up tall ☐		

Initials: _____

FIGURE 12.1   Seating and mobility assessment.

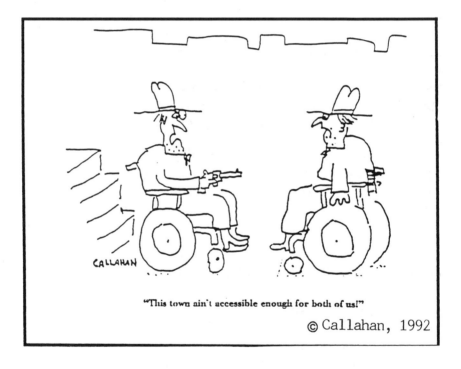

"This town ain't accessible enough for both of us!"

© Callahan, 1992

Optimal Method of Mobility

Legs Only

If a resident is most efficient when using the legs for propulsion, then both feet must reach the ground easily while the pelvis stays back in the chair (see Figures 12.2 and 12.3). To achieve the proper seat-to-floor height, a measurement from the back of the knee to the floor should be taken, making sure to add in the cushion thickness, prior to wheelchair selection or adjustment. Several adjustments can be made to the chair (see Figure 12.4). For instance, a wheelchair can be ordered as a hemi-height chair, which allows seat-to-floor heights to be 2 inches closer to the floor. Also, the wheel size can be altered on certain wheelchairs; instead of the standard 24-inch wheel, a 22- or 20-inch wheel may be necessary to get the resident's feet to the floor with full support. If the rear wheel size is reduced, the front casters will need to be smaller to prevent a downward slant of the seat. The resident's hips should be positioned to the back of the chair with the trunk leaning forward. This will allow for the downward pressure toward the floor that is necessary for forward movement.

It is important to note that if the person is wedged backward into the seat for stability, this will hinder self-mobilization because it is difficult to foot-propel when the hip-to-back angle is decreased. It is actually more efficient to have a flat seat or to angle the seat

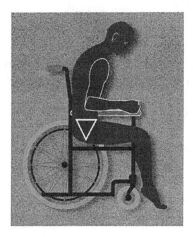

• Feet won't reach floor

FIGURE 12.2   Problem: Propulsion.

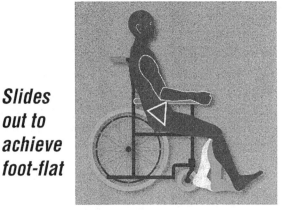

FIGURE 12.3
Problem:
Propulsion.

- *Slides*
  out to
  achieve
  foot-flat

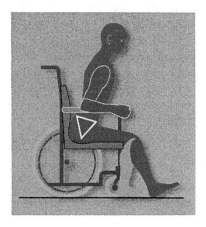

FIGURE 12.4   Solution: Adjust seat-to-floor height.

slightly forward to promote forward movement and also to encourage the trunk to align in a more upright position. Consultation with a seating specialist is recommended for assessment and simulation of seat angles.

Another advantage to having the feet on the floor is that the resident will have the option to rock himself back and forth in the chair. This repetitive motion is not only good for exercising the legs but also provides a calming effect. In addition, when our elderly residents have their feet supported on the ground, they can change not only their foot position but also their pelvic position. We all change our positions often in order to alleviate pain and discomfort by pushing up with our arms and feet. We need to allow residents this opportunity, too.

When residents begin to use their legs more, as a result of good positioning, they are going to be stronger and may attempt to stand, which is a function that should be encouraged. The resident could then be seen by a therapist to determine if upright ambulation is indicated.

Arms-Only Propulsion

When a resident is using both arms, begin by making sure that the wheelchair has the correct width for the size of the person. This is determined by measuring the width of the resident's hips and then selecting a wheelchair width that fits. A rule of thumb is to allow enough space between the hips and the side of the wheelchair for the resident to easily slip his hands between the wheelchair and the hips. The wheelchair width is important because the hand rims should be located in a plumb line under the resident's shoulders. The resident will then be able to achieve the most effective push. A wheelchair that is too wide is therefore difficult to propel.

Once the proper wheelchair width is selected and the feet are fully supported on the footrest without undue pressure under the thighs, then the wheel axle placement needs to be looked at to determine how efficiently the chair can be propelled. For instance, if the rear axis is placed too far behind the resident's vertebral line, the chair will be more stable but the arm motion for pushing will be hindered by inability to reach the wheel for a full push. The optimum placement is directly in line with the vertebral line or slightly behind. This particular adjustment is not always possible on the "standard" wheelchair. If the wheelchair appears too likely to tip backward, adding antitippers to the back of the chair will help.

Other considerations are as follows:

- A small, 20-inch rear wheel may be easier to rotate than a large, 24-inch wheel. When using the arms for mobility, it is important to know that the arms need to move not only forward but also down and backward and then up. This

• *Inadequate Shoulder Extension*

• *Scapular Protraction*

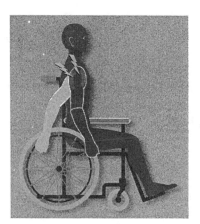

FIGURE 12.5
Unable to propel chair

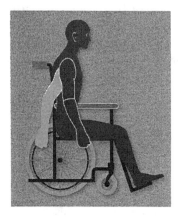

FIGURE 12.6 Solution: Small wheel diameter.

motion will stimulate trunk extension and breathing (see Figures 12.5 & 12.6).

• The hand rims may be easier to grip when covered with a grip-ease material; gloves with leather in the palms are also helpful to create increased friction for propulsion, to keep hands clean, and to protect them from callousing.

• A lightweight wheelchair may be advantageous because it is easier to propel, especially for the elderly, who often have upper extremity weakness.

Combination of One Arm and One Leg

The approach remains the same as those given above, except that the cushion may need to be altered to accommodate one leg being supported on a footrest while the other leg is on the floor. To make this adjustment, a cushion should be considered that can be shortened or scooped out for the thigh of the leg that will be contacting the floor for mobility.

Transfer to and from Wheelchair

If the resident has difficulty getting in and out of the wheelchair, there are several possible solutions.

- Remove or flip up footrests to allow enough space for the resident to place the feet slightly under the wheelchair.
- Remove the armrest that interferes with the resident when he is transferring from the side of the wheelchair to another surface with or without the use of a sliding board.
- Consult a physical therapist for an evaluation to determine the transfer solutions.

Goal 2: Upright Position to Maximize Head and Upper Extremity Function

Assess and Correct Hip or Pelvis Positioning

As mentioned earlier, the most common observation is that the resident's hips are sliding out of the chair. It is important to note that this position can cause a great deal of discomfort. For instance, it can cause low back pain, increased pressure on the sacral area, and poor trunk alignment, which leads to poor head position and a decreased ability to use the upper extremities. Sometimes when a resident has slid forward in the chair, it is because he is trying to reach the floor to use his feet for mobility or to change his position in order to relieve discomfort. But quite often residents are too weak to reposition themselves and become at risk for skin breakdown, slipping out of the chair, and injuring themselves by falling.

When a resident has a thoracic kyphosis and her hips are positioned to the back of the chair, the trunk is pushed forward, and she ends up looking at her lap (see Figure 12.7). She therefore needs to scoot her hips forward in order to have a more level eye gaze. There are several solutions to this problem.

- Attempt to reposition the resident's hips to the back of the chair. If this is not possible, an evaluation is necessary to determine if there are fixed joint limitations, deformities, or muscle tightness.
- If the resident's hips can be relocated to the back of the chair, see that her feet are supported—either flat on the floor or on footrests with light support under the thighs. If the feet are not supported, a simple footrest adjustment may be necessary to support the feet better. A different wheelchair with a lower seat-to-floor height may be indicated for the person who is a foot mobilizer and needs the feet flat on the floor.
- Sometimes a positioning hip belt (either push-button or latch type) is indicated to assist in keeping the hips in the proper place. A hip belt would not be a restraint if the resident wishes to use it and can take it off at will. However, if the resident cannot remove the hip belt independently, it would be a physical restraint, and less restrictive interventions should be considered.
- To accommodate for a kyphotic spine, the back of the wheelchair needs to be reclined enough to allow for the deformity without compromising pelvic positioning.

- *Thoracic Kyphosis*

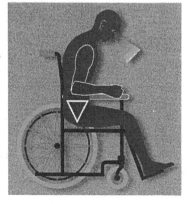

FIGURE 12.7
Problem: Forward lean.

- It may be useful to consult with a specialist for proper trunk placement, alignment for function, and appropriate choice of equipment.

Assess and Correct Equipment (Seating)

Another problem is the effects of sling seating. This type of seating does not provide a level base to position the pelvis and thighs in good alignment. Instead it tends to roll the residents' legs inward and support the buttocks or thighs unevenly. Many older wheelchairs have sling upholstery that is overslung, increasing the hammocking effect and causing pain, discomfort, and sitting intolerance. As mentioned earlier, sling seating was intended for transportation purposes and to allow folding of the wheelchair, not for long-term sitting as occurs with most nursing home residents. There are two ways to address this problem.

1. Sling seating can be replaced with solid seating. Some solid seats are adjustable and can be dropped in order to lower the seat-to-floor height; some also can be adjusted to angle the seat backward or forward to achieve an upright pelvis and position it back in the seat.
2. A solid seat insert can be added across or between the seat rails of a wheelchair that has sling seating. Most solid seat inserts can be placed under the cushion or inside the cushion cover; this consolidates the pieces and may prevent improper placement. A cushion over the solid seat insert is needed for comfort and positioning.

Once the pelvis is positioned, the hips are in the back of the wheelchair, and the back is supported to achieve upper trunk and head control, then adjust the armrest height to support the forearms comfortably. Unfortunately, many of the wheelchairs used in nursing homes have fixed armrests that cannot be adjusted. Another consideration is the length of the armrests. Full-length armrests will provide greater support to a lap tray. A desk-length armrest will allow the resident to pull up closer to a table or sink, which facilitates activities of daily living.

Goal 3: Minimize Trunk Deformity, Maximize Function

Assess Need for Trunk Support

Once the hips are in the proper position, it is time to observe the trunk. If a resident has poor trunk control, several areas can be affected. The upper extremities feel heavier, and the shoulder range becomes limited, leading to decreased functional ability. Improper trunk position can also affect head position, breathing, swallowing, eye gaze, and socialization.

First, are the hips to the back of the wheelchair? (If not, "Assess and Correct Hip or Pelvis Positioning," above.) Once the hips are to the back of the chair, observe the trunk position. Is the resident leaning to one side or is he falling forward? Usually, leaning is caused by weakness, upright orientation problems, or improper pelvis positioning (see Figure 12.8). Installing a lap tray to assist the resident in obtaining an upright position is *not* the appropriate use of a lap tray. The enormous pressure placed on the arms and shoulder joints can cause pain, skin breakdown, and shoulder joint limitation over a long period of time. Also, fatigue occurs from trying to hold up one's trunk weight with one's arms. If a resident needs trunk support, try one of these solutions (see Figure 12.9).

- The pelvis can be positioned level and upright on a firm seating surface against a firm back.
- A slight recline in the back of the wheelchair can decrease the gravitational pull and allow more trunk support. This can be accomplished by replacing the existing back upholstery of the wheelchair with a contoured back that can recline slightly or by using a wheelchair with a reclining back.
- Side trunk supports may be necessary to assist a weak trunk. The side support can be attached to the side of the wheelchair or can be ordered as an option with the back portion of a seating system. A three-point system can be utilized for placement of the lateral supports to maintain trunk alignment.

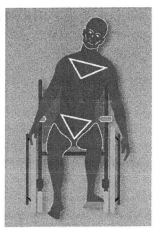

FIGURE 12.8   Problem: Asymmetry.

• *Weakness*
• *Positioning*

• *Firm level base*
• *Lateral support*
• *3-point system*

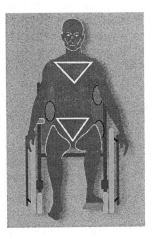

FIGURE 12.9
Solution: Provide support.

• Sometimes trunk weakness is severe enough to require a combination of a reclining back and a side support to allow adequate trunk support for proper positioning and improved functioning.

Remember: the pelvis is the starting point. Make sure the pelvis is properly positioned before attempting to support the trunk. If problems persist or equipment options are unknown, consult a seating specialist.

Goal 4: Minimize Abnormal Foot Position

Assess Foot Position

Feet need to be properly supported in order to maintain the position of the pelvis (keeping the hips to the back of the chair) and to have effective mobility. The wheelchair footrests, for instance, are used to support the feet, but they may not be adjusted high enough or low enough to enhance function and positioning. A change in the position of the feet or pressure felt on the feet can negatively affect the trunk and pelvis position. For instance, if the footrests are too high, the thighs are inadequately supported, and more pressure is placed on the ischial tuberosities, which may lead to discomfort and/or skin breakdown. If the footrests are too low, there is too much pressure on the thighs, and circulatory problems can occur, as well as skin breakdown. If the footrests are placed too far out or if elevating leg rests are used, the resident may scoot out toward the edge of the wheelchair to decrease the stretch on tight hamstrings. If the resident is a foot mobilizer and the seat is too high, he may scoot out to the edge of the chair to get the full foot support needed to achieve efficient and successful mobility.

First, make sure the pelvis is all the way back in the wheelchair because this affects the position of the feet. Then try one of these solutions to the problem.

1. Depending on the wheelchair, the footrests can be adjusted by loosening the bolt at the end of the footrest hanger. If the footrests cannot be adjusted to the proper height, a different wheelchair may be indicated.

2. If the angle of the footrest hangers needs to be altered because of hamstring limitations, another set can be ordered if available, or a solid footplate can be reversed and attached with brackets to the footrests (see Figure 12.10). This supports the feet while providing the knee flexion needed to allow the tight hamstrings some slack. Now the hamstrings no longer pull the pelvis forward at their origin: the ischial tuberosities.

3. If the resident cannot reach the floor without full foot contact for mobilization, the seat can be replaced with a solid drop seat to decrease the seat-to-floor height and allow better floor

- *Feet on floor*
- *<70° foot plate*

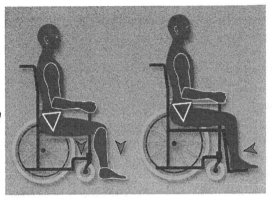

FIGURE 12.10   Solution: Proper foot placement.

contact. A hemi-height wheelchair designed for persons who need to use their feet for mobility can also be considered. The hemi-height chair can be used in combination with a dropped seat, allowing for the seat cushion thickness, which could add 2–4 inches to the seat-to-floor height. If the wheelchair is still not low enough, then it may be necessary to use a smaller wheel size, such as a 22- or 20-inch wheel, and a smaller caster wheel, to lower the chair closer to the floor. Very short residents who need to reach the floor will sometimes need to use a combination of a hemi-height wheelchair and a dropped seat and smaller wheels to achieve the proper seat-to-floor height. This is referred to as a super-hemi-wheelchair. If it is difficult to make the proper adjustments, a seating specialist should be consulted.

Goal 5: Maximize Head Control to Facilitate Interaction with the Environment

Assess the Need for Head Support

Once the hips and trunk are positioned properly, the head should be positioned properly too. In the case of weakness, proper head support is necessary for level eye gaze, orientation, and socialization. If the head is still leaning too far forward, backward, or to one side, an assessment is necessary.

If the resident appears to have poor head control, a headrest, along with a reclined back, could be considered. A more sophisticated seating system may be required, and a seating specialist should be consulted.

Goal 6: Prevent Skin Breakdown

Pressure sores can be caused by improper seating arrangements and/or prolonged sitting, especially among residents who have poor sensation and are unable to reposition themselves. It is important to check the buttocks and back for persistent redness (lasting longer than 20 minutes) and any open skin areas. If residents have existing open sores, they will need special attention to sit in a wheelchair. Here are three approaches to preventing pressure sores.

1. Always check skin thoroughly after transferring the resident from the wheelchair. Pay close attention to the ischial tuberosities, sacrum, coccyx, and spinous processes.
2. When a resident is beginning to use a wheelchair, start slowly until a tolerance has built up for wheelchair sitting. This is especially necessary for the cognitively impaired resident who cannot tell you what is wrong and cannot reposition himself.
3. Pressure-relief cushions are available for wheelchairs. This type of cushion will allow the resident to sit with minor open skin areas or sensitive skin that is susceptible to skin breakdown. Again, constant skin monitoring is necessary to ensure that healing is promoted. A good pressure-relieving cushion needs to be used in combination with regular pressure relief such as shifting weight off of buttocks.

Goal 7: Achieve Reasonable Wheelchair Tolerance— Approximately 6–8 Hours

It is important to note the resident's wheelchair tolerance: How long does she sit in the chair, and what are her reasons for wanting to get out of the chair?

If agitation, irritability, crying, or asking to go back to bed are observed, the resident is probably uncomfortable and cannot tolerate sitting any longer. Long periods of sitting, especially when one is unable to move, may cause increased pressure on bony prominences, which in turn may lead to discomfort, pain, and skin breakdown because of decreased circulation to the skin areas.

To solve this problem, decrease the amount of time the resident spends in the chair or allow frequent rests out of the wheelchair until a more thorough assessment can be done to determine the reason for the resident's intolerance. Many times it is the seating arrangement, and a seating consultant may need to assist with the evaluation and equipment selection in order to increase wheelchair tolerance and decrease pain, discomfort, and decubitus risk.

EQUIPMENT

Currently most nursing homes are expected to provide wheelchairs and walkers for their clients. Many wheelchairs in nursing homes are in constant disrepair. Some facilities employ independent services to repair these chairs and keep them useful for as long as possible. At present, Medicare does not routinely pay for individualized wheelchairs for persons who reside in nursing facilities. State Medicaid offices also often deny funding for seating and mobility devices for elderly nursing home residents. This complicates the nursing home's ability to provide appropriate seating. Medicare and Medicaid does pay for individualized wheelchairs for elderly persons residing in their own home or foster care. Medicaid usually does cover the cost of individualized seating for younger clients. This distinction based on age or where the person resides seems out of date and discriminatory. As we remove restraints from nursing home residents, it becomes clear that we have been tying residents to improper chairs to make the wheelchair "work," while immobilizing the resident and compromising his/her comfort and independence. It appears that new state and federal policies are necessary to address the seating and mobility needs of elderly nursing home residents if they are to reach their highest possible level of function.

Wheelchairs in general should be prescribed for individual needs; one type of wheelchair will not fit all clients. We are all different sizes and shapes, and we all have different functional and mobility needs. A wheelchair needs to accommodate a variety of these needs. It is very unfortunate when a resident has been issued a wheelchair with squeaky wheels that pulls to the left, with wheel locks that do not work, and with upholstery that is torn. This is a sad yet typical problem with wheelchairs in most nursing homes. Every person deserves to have a chair that is appropriate for her particular needs and wants. Wheelchair companies are now trying to individualize wheelchairs by designing chairs with adjustments and options. Residents have places to go and things to do; whether that means from their room to the hallway or out in the community, those options should be available. Mobility allows choices to persons living in a nursing home and improves quality of life.

Selection of Equipment

Seating systems should be the initial focus; solid seating is indicated to distribute pressure, decrease the hammocking effect from

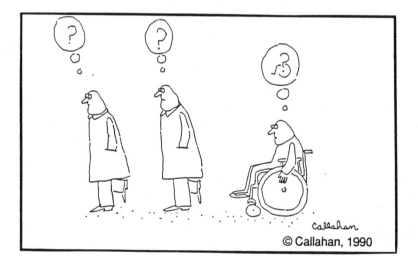

© Callahan, 1990

sling seating, and to allow easier transfers in and out of the wheel-chair. Contouring and padding in seats and backs are also needed, to distribute pressure, alleviate skin breakdown, promote comfort, and increase sitting tolerance. The result may be a decrease in nursing demands. The seating arrangement is crucial for function as well as comfort. In addition, the wheelchair selected can make all the difference in ease of mobility, efficiency of mobility, and stability of the chair for seating.

There are a variety of wheelchairs available. A lightweight wheelchair is the best selection for most older residents because of their upper extremity weakness and inability to efficiently propel a standard-weight wheelchair. Power mobility should not be overlooked for the residents who cannot mobilize themselves. With power capabilities many clients can skillfully maneuver themselves around the nursing home and in the community, given adequate cognition and safety awareness.

Facilities should be upgrading their wheelchair fleets not only to durable wheelchairs but also to lightweight and adjustable wheelchairs. They should have armrest and footrest adjustments to accommodate several different sizes and provide proper support. Adjustments at the wheel axle will assist residents to propel themselves more efficiently. Also, adjusting seat-to-floor height to allow the feet to touch the ground assures foot mobility and support. Some wheelchairs have the option of a slight recline up to 15 degrees in the seat-to-back angle to accommodate kyphosis or support a weak trunk. It is recommended that the hemi-height wheelchair be the standard issue for nursing homes.

It is important to familiarize yourself with the current types of wheelchairs and accessories in order to make the proper selection for your residents. It may be necessary to begin by removing the current sling upholstery from the facility wheelchair and replacing it with dropped solid seats and contoured padding until the mobility base can be replaced by a newer, more versatile, and durable lightweight wheelchair model. There are several commercially available cushion systems that can replace existing upholstery and allow a lower seat-to-floor height.

Care and Maintenance

Ongoing staff in-services that include all nursing home staff are necessary for education on the proper use and maintenance of wheelchair equipment and accessories. It is also necessary to point out the positioning that is being achieved as well as the functional advantages of proper positioning. If a staff member is not trained about the resident's particular maintenance and positioning program, items could be lost or misplaced or not applied correctly.

CONCLUSION

Residents in a nursing home should have a seating evaluation if a wheelchair is indicated. Observation plays a major part in this; you can simply stand in a nursing home and observe how residents are sitting and whether they look comfortable or not. Also, you can observe how the residents are moving or not moving in their wheelchairs. The nursing staff is very important in the observation process and the initiation of an assessment.

It is important that residents be given the opportunity to change their position. We all sit in several different chairs all day. We have a chair that we sit in for eating, we have a chair we sit in when we work, we have a chair we sit in when we drive; we have several chairs we sit in throughout the day, and they are all different. It is important within the nursing home that residents also have alternative seating available to them, such as a recliner for rest and a chair to sit in for mealtime in addition to the wheelchair used for mobility. Also, some residents need to lie down to rest during the day. The wheelchair does not have to be used all day.

ACKNOWLEDGMENT

A special thanks to Antje Hunt, PT; Barbara Riley, KT; Tom Hetzel, PT; and Dee-Dee Freney, OTR, for technical review.

REFERENCE

Shaw, C. G., & Taylor, S. J. (1992). A survey of wheelchair seating problems of the institutionalized elderly. *Assistive Technology, 3*(1), 5–10.

Chapter 13

USE OF SKILLFUL, CREATIVE PSYCHOSOCIAL INTERVENTIONS

Joanne Rader

Learning to communicate with persons suffering from dementia is a key factor in using skillful and creative psychosocial interventions. It is essential that staff be given training and opportunities to practice verbal and nonverbal communication skills. There are a number of very fine videotapes available to help educate staff (see "Resource List," Appendix F).

COMMUNICATING WITH THE RESIDENT

Residents with dementia often have decreased verbal abilities and difficulty in understanding the meaning of what is said to them. However, they are very sensitive to the nonverbal behavior of their caregivers. The staff's attitudes and mood are felt immediately.

The following are helpful nonverbal skills. A slow, calm approach works best; also, approach from the front, not from the side or behind. Looking directly at residents when speaking and establishing eye contact focuses their attention. It is helpful to assume an equal or lower position, especially if the resident feels powerless. Verbal and nonverbal messages need to match, since residents are more inclined to respond to nonverbal messages.

Similarly, caregivers' actions need to be congruent with their promises, to maintain trust and a sense of security.

Verbal communication should consist of precise, positive words or simple sentences delivered in a slow, calm, low voice. Ask one question at a time and wait for a response. Never argue or try to reason. Say exactly what you want residents to do and avoid saying what you do not want them to do. For example, it is easier for a confused resident to follow the command "Stay in the building" than "Don't go outside." Because persons with dementia respond to concrete rather than abstract meanings of words, saying exactly what is intended is also important. One nursing assistant told of asking a woman to "come over and hop into bed." The woman walked to the bed, tried to hop, and turned to the aide to say, "I can't!"

Use both verbal and nonverbal cues when assisting residents to perform activities of daily living. These cues should be geared to their level of functioning and attention span. For example, some residents can brush their teeth if handed a toothbrush in the bathroom. In this case, the visual cue triggers a remembered habit. Others require step-by-step instructions, such as "Move the brush to your mouth; brush up and down," accompanied by a visual demonstration of the process. Instructions need to be given in a consistent manner from one occasion to the next.

Distraction can be used to dissuade a resident with memory impairments from engaging in undesirable activities or responses. For example, if a resident resists preparation for bed, cooperation may be elicited if the caregiver leaves and then returns in 5 minutes. Often the first request will have been forgotten during the short time interval. Similarly, a resident may be distracted from rummaging through another person's possessions by engaging him in a simple task such as dusting or sweeping.

Orienting information, such as calendars and reality-orientation boards, may be helpful to residents in the early stages of dementia. As the disease progresses, however, it is more useful to orient residents to their caregiver and daily tasks than to the date and place. If a woman insists she has been busy all morning doing the wash and getting the children ready for school, compliment her on what a good worker she is instead of correcting her or orienting her to the unit.

Responding to the underlying meaning of what a confused resident wants rather than to the specific words enables the caregiver to identify and address unmet needs or concerns while maintaining the dignity of the resident. Acknowledge the person's feelings and help her "name" them if she has difficulty. Here is an example of this: "You look sad. Do you miss your daughter after she leaves?" Also, identify symbolic behaviors and their meaning. For example, the cup the resident wishes to hang onto after meals may symbolize having coffee with friends and relatives and thus may serve as a source of security and comfort.

AGENDA BEHAVIOR

An important psychosocial concept that can guide interventions is agenda behavior. Agenda behavior is the plan of action and behavior that the cognitively impaired client uses in an attempt to meet his felt social, emotional, or physical needs at a given time (Rader, Doan, & Schwab, 1985). This is a particularly useful concept when dealing with wandering behavior and resistance to care activities.

It is generally best not to thwart a resident's agenda or plan of action, such as wanting to leave the facility to see his mother. Rather, look for the unmet need the resident is expressing and try to meet it in an appropriate way. For instance, requests to go home often represent a desire of residents to find a state of mind where they felt comfortable, secure, loved, or needed rather than a desire to go to a particular geographic location. You can often help create that state of mind by interacting with residents skillfully. Responding to a resident's request to go see her mother by asking her to tell you about her mother, in a sense brings her mother to her.

Mary White, an 83-year-old widow with moderate-to-severe chronic dementia, was admitted to the nursing home, and 4 days later, during the evening meal, she was making a third attempt to leave the building "to fix supper for my children and husband." A nurse approached Mrs. White from behind, took her arm, and said, "This is your home now, Mrs. White; your children are all grown." Mrs. White loudly denied this and struck out at the nurse, who called for help. Two staff members responded, and the three physically returned Mrs. White to her chair and applied a vest restraint. She continued to yell and pulled on the restraint, overturning her meal tray and striking at anyone who approached. The nurse telephoned Mrs. White's physician, who prescribed a tranquilizer.

This sequence of events is not uncommon in some long-term care facilities. Mary White's agenda was to go home and prepare supper. She was merely disoriented and restless at the start of the interaction. Underlying her attempt to leave the facility was a need to feel connected with people (family) and to be of service. The staff, by ignoring Mary White's emotions and needs and by thwarting her plan, increased her agitation and thus precipitated her combative behavior.

An alternative method of handling Mrs. White's behavior would have been to approach her from the front, establish eye contact, and repeat what she had said, thus acknowledging her emotional need and reinforcing it. You, the nurse, could say, "Mrs. White, you need to fix dinner for your family? I bet you are a good cook and took good care of your family. Are you worried?" This reflection of her feelings lets the individual know she's been heard and understood and is thus in full touch with another person. (Even if a patient is dysphasic and using jargon, repeating a portion of the jargon is necessary to evoke the feeling of being connected with another person; that is what the resident must sense if she is to feel safe and decide to stay.)

Continuing to talk about Mrs. White's family, you might gently take her arm and guide her away from the door. If unable to distract her from leaving the building, follow her out, continuing the conversation. Her limited attention span and the sense of connectedness and security increasing between you and Mrs. White may allow you, in a short time, to redirect her to the building.

Provide orienting information only if she requests it or if it helps. "Correcting" often makes the individual feel more separate and wrong. If you cannot immediately redirect her, continue to walk with her, letting her choose the direction but protecting her safety as needed.

There are two expected outcomes of this alternative intervention. The cognitively impaired person's agenda or need for it will play itself out over time as that person feels more listened to and more connected with someone. Agitation and combativeness will subside and thus the need for physical or pharmaceutical restraint.

If all of the staff in the nursing home (dietary staff, housekeepers, administrators, and volunteers, as well as nurses) are taught to use good verbal and nonverbal communication techniques, most "problem" behaviors can be prevented. Some individuals have a natural understanding of how to communicate with persons with dementia. Others can be taught. A few seem incapable of learning or altering their own style to accommodate the needs of residents. These staff members, who may be consistently loud, anxious, rushed, task-oriented, controlling, and abrupt, will frequently precipitate catastrophic reactions and excess disability in residents. They often lack insight into how their behaviors affect others. Supervisors and administrators need to be sure that attitudes and approaches to care are a documented part of the routine evaluation of staff so that if these behaviors persist in spite of role modeling, education, and direct supervision, there is a mechanism for informing staff members that they are not suited for this line of work and should seek other employment. If that does not work, they should be fired. To continue to employ staff members who have consistently poor psychosocial skills with residents creates more work for others and severely limits the quality of life for residents.

REFERENCE

Rader, J., Doan, J., & Schwab, M. (1985). How to decrease wandering, a form of agenda behavior. *Geriatric Nursing, 6*(4), 196–199.

Chapter 14

ACTIVITY INTERVENTIONS

Doris Weaver

OVERVIEW

> Activity of some kind, whether it's work or play, active or passive, exciting or mundane, is to most people synonymous with living. It is the way in which each person defines himself and his role in society and exerts control over the world around him. (Zgola, 1987)

The challenge to staff working with the cognitively impaired resident is to view activities as more than a recreational or social event. Most older persons have spent their lives being productive, working at daily tasks, responding to the needs of those around them, and occasionally playing. Older persons who no longer have the opportunity to experience a feeling of being needed and productive have lost their familiar roles, social identity, and purpose. It is essential that activity programming for persons with dementia be a part of a therapeutic activity program that maximizes remaining functions, enhances quality of life, and validates each individual

While developing the activity program, remember that the aim is to enhance the quality of life of each resident. There are tremendous emotional and behavioral consequences when a person feels devalued or is devalued by those around him. The goals of an activity program for the cognitively impaired, therefore, must be to

197

define social roles, reduce feelings of failure, provide a sense of inclusion and belonging, and enhance self-esteem.

An activity program that accomplishes these goals can provide positive social, cognitive, emotional, and behavioral outcomes for each person involved.

THE MAGICIAN'S ROLE

In the story *The Velveteen Rabbit* by Margery Williams, a child's nursery is filled with toys that have been discarded in favor of newer ones. The Rabbit, who has been "shelved," asks the old and worn Skin Horse, "What's real? Does it mean having things that buzz inside you and a stick-out handle?"

"Real isn't how you are made," says the Skin Horse. "It's a thing that happens to you. When a child loves you for a long time, not just to play with you but REALLY loves you, then you become Real." As in *The Velveteen Rabbit*, so it is in real life—caring and loving create magic.

Our challenge is to look beyond the physical and cognitive changes that have "shelved" people and dulled their responses. To work magic, we must have a special understanding of residents. The magician's job includes

- gaining insight into the special emotional needs of the resident
- identifying the resident's remaining strengths
- understanding what is meaningful and provides satisfaction to the resident

There are a variety of ways to do this, including experiential exercises, simulating sensory losses, developing a biographical sketch, and listing strengths and needs.

Experiential Exercises

It is always difficult to understand the needs of another person. It is not surprising, then, that it is a challenge for staff and families to understand the emotional and behavioral needs of residents. Experiential exercises can be used to sensitize caregivers to the emotional impact of physical and cognitive loss of control.

Sensory losses increase as persons grow older. Sensory impairment simulation can provide insight into the feelings and emotions that often result and that may be exhibited as undesirable behaviors. Provide staff with eyeglasses, earplugs, gloves, and taped fingers, then ask them to participate in several typical activities used in your programs (see Appendix G). After the exercise, discuss their responses—what were they feeling emotionally and physically? How did they behave or want to behave?

Another useful exercise (Zgola, 1990) is to provide the staff with two pieces of paper. Ask them to list on one all the exciting recreational things they like to do. On the other, ask them to list all the regular and mundane things they do throughout the day. When they finish, ask them to hold one list in each hand and take an imaginary walk down the street. Suddenly they will meet the Grim Reaper, who says, "Your time is up. However, I will give you another 20 years if you will give me one of the lists in your hand. Think carefully, for once you've given me the list, you will never do those things again!" Give the group time to think and discuss.

- Which list would you give up?
- What would it mean to you?
- Where are the greater rewards in life?
- What provides self-esteem?
- Could you participate in and enjoy recreational activities if you could not do the things on the other list?

Understanding the Resident

The most telling and most useful information about a resident is sometimes found in the past. A skilled activity staff will ask questions of family, friends, the minister, and others who have known the resident for years. Being aware of overlearned patterns, past coping skills, and values is essential. Despite deficits, many residents retain important strengths that, when supported, can make activities a more positive experience.

When a person has dementia, it is essential to go beyond the traditional information gathering at admission. Care plans, activities, and behavioral interventions are much more effective when we know about overlearned patterns (such as folding clothes, dancing, setting tables, etc.), past coping skills and past—rather than current—interests. Some nursing homes have found it helpful to send a letter to the family asking them to write a biographical sketch, based on memories of 20 to 40 years ago (see Table 10.3, for example). This information is invaluable in developing not only activity programs but the entire therapeutic approach to the resident. A number of facilities have reported increased self-esteem for residents and increased socialization between residents and between staff and residents when Bioboards were placed on the hall by each resident's door.

It is sometimes difficult to discover the needs and remaining strengths of a person who is physically or cognitively impaired. The purpose of the exercise described below is to help staff identify the need behaviors may represent and use the strengths that remain in developing a care plan for dealing with behaviors.

You will need a flip chart and two colors of felt-tip pens. Ask one staff person to present a challenging case study to the group. Have the group respond with what they think the needs might be, and list them as they are given. Next ask the group to identify the strengths the person still has (this is more difficult). Then develop a care plan and approach using the information from the first part of the exercise.

THE ROLE OF THE DETECTIVE

An activity staff "magician" must also be a good detective. The detective's job is to find clues to successful activities. Persons with dementia present a challenge to those planning activities. Looking for clues in the following areas can be helpful: psychosocial needs, common areas of dysfunction, and emotional needs.

It is important to be aware that the person with dementia continues to experience psychological and social needs. When attempting to understand psychological strengths and deficits, it is necessary to assess the resident's past and current coping styles. The following are basic psychosocial needs: need for identity, need for control and independence, and need for self-esteem.

Successful activities for the cognitively impaired require understanding the limitations of the resident because of the gradual changes in the brain due to disease. With understanding, the staff can make adaptations that will reduce the chances of failure and meet the emotional needs of the resident. Activity planning should take into consideration dysfunctions in memory, perception, organization of movement, language, judgment, and abstraction.

Memory

Short-term memory loss is the inability to learn new things, with associated difficulty in staying attentive. For residents with memory problems, choose a quiet area for small groups and one-to-one activities, provide one-step instructions, and rely on remote memory for interactions.

Perception Dysfunction

Agnosia (distorted perception) interferes with the person's ability to interpret stimuli accurately. This can cause the resident to misunderstand visual, auditory, and tactile cues.

For residents with agnosia, always identify objects, use visual cues, and demonstrate tasks.

Organization of Movement

Apraxia is the inability to organize and sequence specific tasks on command. To deal with this, lay out objects in an appropriate sequence, and try using music to initiate movement.

Language

Language problems are common and frustrating to the resident. They include inability to find the right word, misuse of words, and talking "around" the subject.

When a resident has language problems, listen for "key" words and watch the nonverbal language. Demented persons continue to express themselves in many ways beyond words.

Judgment

Judgment problems include the inability to anticipate problems and make appropriate choices. Therefore it may be necessary at times to limit choices. For example, instead of asking the individual what she wants to eat, it may be better to know her preferences and state, "Here's some mashed potatoes; I know you like them."

Abstraction

Difficulty in forming abstract concepts prevents the resident from being able to visualize stories or objects unless given concrete tactile or visual cues. Therefore, always use some type of visual aid when telling stories (flannel board, pictures, objects). Eliminate multiple-choice selections.

Emotional Needs

Every resident, in spite of physical and cognitive deficits, deserves to be recognized as a unique individual with emotional needs. For the person with dementia, the day is often filled with mistakes, obstacles, and failures. The role of the detective is to identify the needs of the resident that are not being met and use that information to develop activities and programs. The observant detective will look for cues in the following areas of emotional need: for loving and being loved, for inclusion, for quiet times, for socialization, for reassurance, for acceptance, for praise, and for recognition.

THE ROLE OF THE CARPENTER

Years wrinkle the skin but to give up enthusiasm wrinkles the soul.—Author unknown

A carpenter has a vision of what it will take to build the activity program needed to enhance the quality of life for each resident. A good carpenter enthusiastically gathers every conceivable tool that is appropriate for the various levels of functioning and unique needs of residents. The carpenter sees challenges and uses appropriate tools to obtain desired results. To ensure adequate opportunities for participation in activities that offer reasonable success, the following types of activities have been suggested (Helm & Wekstein, 1991).

Types of Activities

- Mental Stimulation: Any activity that promotes exercise of the mind. Examples: reading, conversation, games, reminiscence.
- Socialization: Any activity that promotes interaction with one or more other individuals. Examples: meals, discussion groups, parties.
- Creative Activity: Any activity that promotes the individual's ability to create something that is meaningful and unique. Examples: arts and crafts, poetry, storytelling, music.
- Productive Activity: Any activity that promotes the individual's sense of self-worth and meaning. Examples: daily chores, building something, providing a service to another.
- Emotionally Supportive Activity: Any activity that promotes the person's sense of well-being, security, and trust. Examples: support group, counseling, one-to-one attention.
- Physical Activity: Any activity that promotes physical health and mobility. Examples: exercise, walking, music, and movement.
- Personal Care: Any activity that involves daily personal health and hygiene. Examples: bathing, dressing, grooming, and eating.

Within each category there are many creative ways to develop group and one-to-one activity programs for residents. Groups should be kept small except for music and dancing. Even then, some older persons will be overstimulated, so careful observance of tolerance level is needed. Following are a few suggested tools for use in activity planning.

Music

Music is a universal language that promotes responses that are therapeutic for the resident. However, music that is familiar to the resident is best. Several tapes have been developed specifically for the nursing home population (see "Resource List" in Appendix F). Music has these effects:

- Increases alertness.
- Encourages movement.
- Reduces anxiety.
- Relaxes.
- Provides inclusion.
- Facilitates speech.
- Facilitates reminiscence.

Storytelling

Storytelling is a wonderful opportunity for laughter, sharing, and warmth. Because the person with dementia does not have the ability to create visual images with the voice alone, it is important to provide visual, tactile, or olfactory cues such as flannel boards (see "Resource List," Appendix F), pictures, and objects to touch (an old Ball canning jar).

These can help stimulate memories and "create" the moment. We learn to "celebrate the temporary."

Reminiscence

Reminiscence is a way to validate the "being" of the older person and a way for the person to say, "I have a history." Reminiscence has these benefits:

- Improves quality of life and well-being, improves self-esteem.
- Heals loneliness and isolation.
- Helps in coping with grief or loss.
- Gives a sense of continuity.
- Helps the person find meaning and purpose in life.
- Provides intergenerational understanding

Physical Activity

Exercise is a very necessary tool, but it is often the least creative activity. The inventive carpenter will include

- planned walking
- dance therapy
- rhythmic movement
- music and creative movement
- unison stretch exercises
- storytelling exercises (tell a story while leading residents with accompanying movements)

And More Tools

Refer to the resident's biographical sketch and explore ways of using residual skills. Make activities an opportunity to celebrate remaining strengths. Explore

- art therapy
- household chores (folding baby clothes, matching socks, raking leaves, sweeping)
- cooking
- business skills (file folders with papers, school paper for teachers to correct).

When working with residents with dementia, we continue to be challenged by behaviors that communicate anxiety and distress. Our goals must be to respond to emotional discomfort in the resident, prevent a catastrophic response, and decrease the use of physical and chemical restraints. When we use appropriate one-to-one activities, residents can be diverted, engaged, and then quietly left with something to keep them engaged. An observant staff person will notice when a resident is becoming anxious, quickly assess the need, and respond with some appropriate "tool" to meet that need. Skill in this process can prevent catastrophic reactions.

For example, Mrs. Watson had been quietly walking the hallway when an observant staff member became aware that she was walking a little faster and beginning to wring her hands. The staff person quietly walked with her and guided her to a quiet area and gently massaged her hands while singing softly. The staff person then gently placed a soft, tactile object in Mrs. Watson's hands, initiated a stroking motion, and left.

Mr. Beck may provide another illustration. He was sitting in the hallway in a wheelchair with a tray and began to yell. A staff person took a "tool box" (a small plastic tackle box with recognizable male items (hinges, PVC joints, locks, etc.) to him and quietly opened it, took things out, and said, "George, will you fix my tool box?" He then engaged him in the task and quietly left.

CONCLUSIONS

Developing activity programs for the cognitively impaired requires sensitive understanding of the cognitive, physical, and emotional needs of each resident. The staff must have an awareness of each person, the person's history, and the significance of that information in planning activities. The program must be flexible and creative, with the ability to go beyond traditional approaches. Developing activities for the cognitively impaired can be challenging, but the rewards are great.

REFERENCES

Helm, B., & Wekstein, D. (1991). *For those who take care: An Alzheimer's Disease training program for nursing assistants.* Lexington, KY: University of Kentucky, Alzheimer's Disease Research Center.

Zgola, J. (1987). *Doing things.* Baltimore: The Johns Hopkins University Press.

Zgola, J. (1990). Therapeutic activity. In N. Mace (Ed.), *Dementia care: Patient, family, and community.* Baltimore: The Johns Hopkins University Press.

Chapter 15

USING PSYCHOACTIVE MEDICATIONS

William Simonson

AGE-RELATED CHANGE IN MEDICATION DOSAGE REQUIREMENTS

Recently, the use and misuse of antipsychotic medications have received a great deal of attention. Antipsychotic drugs are very powerful medications. When used appropriately, they can be highly effective, restoring a resident's quality of life and independence. However, they are also capable of causing many adverse effects. Of course, this is also true of many other different classes of prescription medications that are not under such scrutiny. One explanation is that most classes of medications are used for reasons that are quite clear. For example:

- Antihypertensives are used to treat high blood pressure.
- Cardiac drugs are used for cardiac problems.
- Antibiotics are used to treat infections.

In contrast, the indicators for use of antipsychotics are less clear. Antipsychotics have historically been used for many reasons in addition to treating psychosis, including agitation, wandering, and insomnia.

Problems with the overuse of the powerful antipsychotic medications have been well documented in nursing homes, and they have resulted in new regulations designed to reduce their inappropriate use. The regulations and numerous articles published on the subject have attempted to clarify when it is appropriate to use antipsychotic medications, as well as when it is inappropriate. However, many health care professionals are still confused about how antipsychotic drugs fit into therapy.

Before discussing specifics related to the use of psychoactive medications, it is important to first discuss some of the age-related changes that make older individuals more susceptible to the ill effects of drugs.

Those of us who work with the elderly are well aware of the fact that an 80-year-old individual is not the same as a 20- or 30-year-old. Many differences are obvious; what is not so obvious are the differences that we should expect from drug therapy in the elderly.

Medications taken by elderly individuals generally work the same as in the young; therefore, we should expect antihypertensives to lower blood pressure (though not necessarily to the 120/80 that we would hope to achieve in a younger individual); we should expect antibiotics to cure infections just as they do in the young; and we expect insulin to lower the blood glucose just as it does in the young.

Just as the aging process affects the external body, changes take place internally that may have an influence on drug therapy. These changes are one focus of a relatively new and growing specialty area of pharmacy called pharmacokinetics—the study of what happens to a medication in the body *after* it is taken.

While a detailed discussion of clinical pharmacokinetics—the science of dosage individualization—is beyond the scope of this chapter, some basic summary points may provide a perspective on the subject.

With aging, gradual but substantial changes occur in physical stature. In general, elderly persons are of smaller physical stature than younger adults. Contributing factors include the loss of muscle mass as well as decreases in height—the result of changes in posture as well as compression of the spinal column due to osteoporosis.

The simple fact that older individuals are, as a rule, smaller than younger people provides a powerful justification for using smaller doses. After all, we do not all wear the same size hats or gloves. Why would anyone assume that we should all require the same dose of medication?

Body composition also changes with age; the percentage of body fat increases, and there is a corresponding decrease in muscle mass and in the percentage of body water. Since most medications are preferentially distributed to either body fat or body water, concentrations of drug in the bloodstream and other tissues in the elderly might differ from those in the young. If a medication is fat-soluble, it may be stored in a person's fatty tissue and released into the bloodstream gradually over a period of time, resulting in a more prolonged effect. On the other hand, a medication that is soluble in water might reach higher concentrations—and therefore have greater effect or toxicity—in an elderly individual who has a lower percentage of water in the body.

Kidney function and liver function gradually decline with age, even in the healthy elderly. Since most medications are eliminated from the body either through metabolism by the liver, excretion by the kidneys, or a combination of the two, these changes can be significant. As drug elimination by these routes decreases, "clearance" from the body also decreases. There is a corresponding increase in the time that it takes for the drug to be eliminated from the body, thus increasing the drug's half-life.

The clinical implications of alterations in body size, composition, and organ function are not entirely clear, and they depend on many variables; however, it is well known that these changes result in decreased dosage requirements for some medications. It is important that elderly patients receive medication dosages tailored to their needs so that we can maximize the therapeutic benefits of drug therapy while avoiding toxicity and adverse reactions.

DEFINITIONS

One source of confusion surrounding the antipsychotics and other psychoactive drugs is in the definitions used. The following are "user-friendly" definitions that can help categorize these medications and assist in identifying when the drug might be considered unnecessary.

Unnecessary Drugs

The *Interpretive Guidelines for Nursing Home Surveyors* stipulate that a resident's drug regimen must be free from unnecessary drugs. Unnecessary drugs are defined (section 483.25, F342–347) as any drug used

- in excessive doses
- for excessive periods of time
- without adequate monitoring
- without adequate indications for its use
- in the presence of adverse consequences that indicate the dose should be reduced or discontinued
- for any combination of the reasons above

Psychoactive Drugs

A psychoactive drug is any medication that affects the psyche—attitude, behavior, or degree of awareness. A wide range of medications—and even nonpharmaceutical products, including the caffeine in coffee and the alcohol in wine—may be considered psychoactive drugs. Figure 15.1 illustrates the major categories of

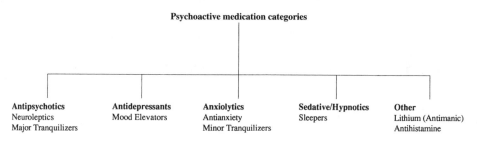

FIGURE 15.1 Psychoactive or psychotropic drug categories commonly used to treat behavioral symptoms.

psychoactive medications. The first name listed under each category represents the most common name used to describe that category. The names below are less common or out-of-date names for the same category.

Antipsychotic Drugs

An antipsychotic is any medication used to treat true psychosis and related conditions, such as distress related to organic mental syndromes. These medications are used for the big problems, such as fearful, distressing hallucinations and delusions. They are also sometimes called "major tranquilizers," although that definition is outdated and infrequently used. Antipsychotics include medications such as

- Haldol (haloperidol)
- Mellaril (thioridazine)
- Thorazine (chlorpromazine)

Antipsychotics have received a great deal of attention, most of it negative, from medical journals, articles in popular magazines, and even Ann Landers. Much of this "bad press" is justified, but most of the problems commonly associated with antipsychotic drugs are not caused by the drugs but by their inappropriate use—for example, for too long a period, at too high a dose, in the wrong patient, or for the wrong reason.

Antidepressants

Antidepressants are medications used to treat depression. As depression resolves, the patient progresses back to a baseline normal, nondepressed state. In the past, antidepressants were sometimes called mood elevators. This term created some misunderstanding about what an antidepressant does—it does not stimulate the mood or make a person "high" or happy; it simply resolves depression. Consequently, the term "mood elevator" is considered outdated and is infrequently used.

Recently, the study of antidepressant use and misuse in the elderly has received a great deal of attention. Some scientific studies have found that depression is very common in the elderly, more common than previously believed, especially in the nursing home. Studies have also demonstrated that antidepressants are often used inappropriately; but unlike antipsychotic medications, which historically have been used too frequently, antidepressant medications are commonly underused, depriving depressed patients of the potential benefits of these medications.

In 1991, the National Institutes of Health published guidelines for the use of antidepressants. Here are just a few of the important points presented in the guidelines:

- Numerous social and physical problems often interfere with proper diagnosis and management of depression in late life.
- Attentive and focused clinical assessment is essential for diagnosis.
- Treatment in depressed elderly should be vigorous, with sufficient doses of antidepressants used for a sufficient length of time.
- Estimates of prevalence of depression vary widely, but prevalence is highest in nursing homes and other residential settings where staff members often are not equipped to recognize or treat depressed patients.

Additional valuable information about the diagnosis and treatment of depression was published in 1993 by the Agency for Health Care Policy Research (AHCPR). The agency emphasized how important it is to consider the adverse drug effects of antidepressant medications. For example, the agency pointed out that the most frequent problems caused by the older antidepressant drugs are anticholinergic effects, because of their ability to block the effects of a neurotransmitter called acetylcholine. These effects commonly include dry mouth, constipation, blurred vision, urinary retention, and occasionally confusion and even hallucinations.

The AHCPR pointed out that many of the newer antidepressants that have become available in the past few years may be as effective as the more traditional agents while causing fewer adverse effects.

Here are a few important points about antidepressant medications:

- Many different antidepressants are available.
- They all treat depression equally well.
- They must be used very carefully in the elderly because they all cause side effects and may interfere with preexisting disease conditions.
- Therapy should be individualized for each patient.
- Therapy should be appropriately aggressive.

The older antidepressants include

- Elavil (amitriptyline)
- Pamelor (nortriptyline)

Newer antidepressants are

- Prozac (fluoxetin)
- Zoloft (sertraline)
- Wellbutrin (bupropion)
- Desyrel (trazadone)

Antianxiety Drugs

Antianxiety medications are used to treat anxiety. They are most commonly represented by the benzodiazepines, such as

- Valium (diazepam)
- Xanax (alprazolam)

There are long- and short-acting benzodiazepines. The long-acting drugs can be dangerous when used with elderly residents since they may cause residual drowsiness and may contribute to an increased incidence of falls.

Historically, the use of antianxiety drugs has not been as problematic as the use of antipsychotics; however, many of the same principles that apply to antipsychotics apply to antianxiety agents.

Since anxiety can be caused by a number of different factors and can vary in severity, there is a potential for inappropriate use of medications to treat this condition. Like the antipsychotic drugs, antianxiety drugs must be used for specific indications. These include

- generalized anxiety disorder
- organic mental syndromes (including dementia) that are quantitatively and objectively documented and constitute sources of distress or dysfunction to the resident or represent a danger to the resident or others
- panic disorder
- symptomatic anxiety that occurs in residents with another diagnosed psychiatric disorder (e.g., depression, adjustment disorder)

Here are a few commonsense guidelines for the appropriate use of antianxiety drugs:

- Try to rule out the cause of the anxiety before considering drug therapy.
- Consider using a nondrug intervention first; it might be more effective than a drug and has no chance of adverse drug side effects.
- Use shorter-acting drugs rather than longer-acting ones.
- Use the medication at a dosage appropriate for the resident.
- Do not use the drug for long periods—more than 4 months—unless attempts have been made to reduce the dosage.
- Use the drug only if it is benefiting the resident by maintaining or improving his functional status.

Anxiolytic Drugs

An anxiolytic is a compound that "lyses" or "breaks" anxiety; thus, it is an antianxiety medication.

Sedatives/Hypnotics

Sedatives or hypnotic medications are often called "sleepers" because they help to induce sleep. The idea of having medications that can safely induce long periods of natural sleep is an attractive one; however, it must be emphasized that the medications currently available do not do that. Some medications that are not true sedative/hypnotics are used as "sleepers" because of their sedative/hypnotic side effects. The antihistamine Benadryl (diphenhydramine) is a good example. When it is used for a runny nose, the drowsiness that commonly occurs with this drug is considered a side effect, especially when one is operating a vehicle. When the drug is used for sleep, the dry nose that it causes might be considered an unwanted, though expected side effect.

Certainly sedatives/hypnotics induce sleep, providing many persons with much-needed rest; however, they are not meant to substitute for real sleep. The sleep-inducing effect of these medications may wear off when they are used routinely. They are also capable of causing a number of serious side effects; longer-acting drugs commonly result in residual drowsiness the morning after their use, contributing to falls. Also, with routine use residents may develop dependence on these drugs. The abrupt discontinuation of these agents after prolonged use may result in a withdrawal reaction characterized by irritability, nervousness, and trouble sleeping, or less frequently, confusion, tachycardia, and trembling. In rare cases withdrawal involves delirium and convulsions. Because of these potential problems it is necessary to avoid prolonged use of these medications.

The most common medications to induce sleep are from the chemical class called benzodiazepines. These and a few other chemical classes of drugs are considered appropriate. Some of the older sedatives/hypnotics, of the class of drugs referred to as barbiturates, are generally considered to be too dangerous to use because of their ability to cause serious depression of the central nervous system.

Shorter-acting benzodiazepines considered appropriate:

- temazepam (Restoril)
- Triazolam (Halcion)

Nonbenzodiazepines considered appropriate:

- chloral hydrate (many brands)
- diphenhydramine (Benadryl)
- zolpidem (Ambien)

Long-acting benzodiazepines not considered appropriate as first-choice drugs:

- flurazepam (Dalmane)
- diazepam (Valium)

Avoid using all barbiturates, including

- pentobarbital (Nembutal)
- phenobarbital (many brands)
- secobarbital (Seconal)

Here are a few commonsense guidelines for the appropriate use of sedatives/hypnotics:

- Try to rule out the cause of the insomnia before considering drug therapy.
- Consider nondrug interventions first; a nondrug intervention might be more effective than a drug, and it has no chance of adverse drug side effects.
- Use shorter-acting drugs rather than longer-acting ones.
- Use the geriatric dose (usually half that of the normal adult dose).
- Use the drug for a short period, less than 10 consecutive days.
- Use the drug only if it benefits the resident by maintaining or improving his functional status.

Antimanic Drugs

Antimanic medications, such as lithium, are used to treat mania.

Medications to Treat Multiple Effects

Keep in mind that definitions are not always absolute. For example, if Mellaril (thioridazine) is used to control psychotic behavior and it also helps the patient sleep because of its sedative properties, is it an antipsychotic, a sedative/hypnotic, or a sedating antipsychotic?

Appendix E, "Psychoactive Medication Information Sheets," gives information about the effects and side effects of each major category of psychoactive medications. The fact sheets give pertinent diagnoses, target symptoms, and a list of commonly used drugs. The fact sheet information can be used to assist in monitoring drug effectiveness and assessing potential drug side effects.

ANTIPSYCHOTIC DRUG USE: A RISK/BENEFIT ANALYSIS

All medications, including antipsychotics, have risks associated with their use as well as benefits. If antipsychotics are to be used, you must consider their potential risks and the appropriate indications for their use. It is critical to be aware of what antipsychotics *are* and what they *are not*, what they are *capable* of doing and what they *cannot* do.

Inappropriate Indications for Antipsychotic Drugs

Antipsychotic drugs should not be used as "chemical restraints." While they may be able to control behavior, using them simply to control behavior cannot be defined as "better living through chemistry." Antipsychotics may control behavior, but they do so by sedating the patient, turning him into a "zombie," not getting to the root of the problem. Using antipsychotics to control behavior in one person for the convenience of someone else is inappropriate and just plain wrong.

Antipsychotic drugs are inappropriate *when these conditions are the only indication for use*:

- Wandering
- Poor self-control
- Restlessness
- Impaired memory
- Anxiety
- Depression
- Insomnia
- Unsociability
- Indifference to surroundings
- Fidgeting
- Nervousness
- Uncooperativeness
- Unspecified agitation

Appropriate Indications for Antipsychotic Drugs

Antipsychotics are indicated for the management of psychosis and psychosis-related disorders. After all, that is why they are called antipsychotics.

A Word in Defense of Antipsychotic Drugs

We must not forget that many people today are able to work and lead high-quality lives primarily because of the benefits that they have experienced from these "miracle drugs." Antipsychotics are not inherently bad, but their inappropriate use is likely to cause serious problems.

Appropriate indications (reasons) for use of these drugs are

- schizophrenia
- schizoaffective disorder
- delusional disorder
- psychotic mood disorders (including mania and depression with psychotic features)
- acute psychotic episodes

- brief reactive psychosis
- schizophreniform disorder
- atypical disorder
- Huntington's disease

Although they are not indicated for the control of simple behavioral symptoms, antipsychotics are appropriate to use for organic mental syndromes, including dementia with associated psychotic and/or agitated features as defined by specific behaviors such as biting, kicking, and scratching, if the specific behavior is quantitatively documented by the facility and if the behavior causes the resident to

- present a danger to self
- present a danger to others, including staff
- interfere with the staff's ability to provide care

Antipsychotics are also used for short-term treatment of

- hiccups
- nausea
- vomiting
- pruritus

Risks of Antipsychotic Therapy

There are risks associated with all drug therapy, and the antipsychotics are certainly no exception. The list of possible adverse effects is long, though some problems are more likely to occur than others. The following adverse drug reactions are directly related to the pharmacology of the drugs (see Table 15.1).

Adverse Effects

Another way to consider adverse consequences is "adverse effects," which are the practical consequences of one or more adverse reactions. Adverse effects may include

Table 15.1 Antipsychotic Medication Adverse Drug Reactions

Central nervous system	Autonomic nervous system blockade	Cholinergic blockade	Tardive dyskinesia
Sedation Depression Extrapyramidal Dystonia/dyskinesia Akathisia Parkinsonian (akinesia, tremor, rigidity	Adrenergic blockade Orthostatic hypotension	Dry mouth Blurred vision Sexual dysfunction Aggravation of narrow angle Glaucoma Urinary retention Constipation Tachycardia	Abnormal involuntary movements
Neuroendocrine effects	Allergic Effects	Pigmentation	
Regulation of body temperature Weight gain Galactorrhea/ amenorrhea	Rash/photo- sensitivity	Corneal, lenticular Retinopathy Skin	

- falls and fractures
- loss of contact with the environment
- poorer quality of life

If a resident receiving an antipsychotic drug experiences orthostatic hypotension (a transient lowering of blood pressure, usually experienced when changing from a lying to a standing position), it may only cause a little dizziness or it may result in a fall and catastrophic injury.

If a resident is given an antipsychotic to control dangerously aggressive behavior and winds up lethargic, sedated, and drooling in a wheelchair, the resident has lost contact with his environment. When kicking or hitting, the resident was in contact with the environment, although perhaps too much so. Often, alternative interventions, in conjunction with lower doses of medication, will

Table 15.2 Adverse Reaction Profile For Common Antipsychotics

	EPS*	Sedation	Anticholinergic	Orthostatic hypotension
Haldol (haloperidol)	+ + + +	+	+	+
Thorazine (chlorpromazine)	+ +	+ + +	+ + +	+ + +
Mellaril (thioridazine)	+	+ + +	+ + + +	+ + +

* Extra-pyramidal Syndrome = Parkinsonian-like tremors, rigidity, drooling, mask-like face.
Adapted from Drug Regimen Review: A Process Guide for Pharmacists, 1992 American Society of Consultant Pharmacists, Alexandria VA.

successfully decrease those behaviors; excessive doses that create sedation are not needed.

Certain adverse effects are more likely to be associated with particular antipsychotic medications. Knowing the most likely adverse effects can help guide the prescriber to the proper choice of antipsychotic medication. Table 15.2 demonstrates some differences between the most commonly used antipsychotic medications.

Since haloperidol (Haldol) is less likely than other drugs to cause sedation, this drug might be most appropriate when you want to avoid sedation, for example, in the case of a resident who is actively involved in recreational or occupational therapy. On the other hand, thioridazine (Mellaril) has a greater sedative effect and might be the most appropriate medication for a resident who is agitated and cannot sleep.

ASSESSMENT OF ANTIPSYCHOTIC THERAPY

Goal of Therapy

Appropriate antipsychotic use can be encouraged by thoroughly considering the risks and benefits of therapy in a particular resident.

Antipsychotics are not for the treatment of simple wandering; they are not "antiwandering drugs"; they are not "anti–poor self-care drugs" or "antirestlessness drugs"; and they are not for "dementia," "senility," or "old age." They are antipsychotics. When behavioral problems are the direct result of a psychosis-related condition or when they are serious, the use of antipsychotics is appropriate as long as the resident's behavior is documented and quantified.

The risks of antipsychotic therapy, which are many, must be considered with each resident. If the potential benefits exceed the risks, then the decision to initiate therapy may be appropriate. Prior to initiating antipsychotic therapy, the prescriber, all caregivers, and the resident and family should understand the desired goals. These goals must represent realistic expectations and be quantifiable so that the degree of success in achieving the goals can be determined (see Appendix A, Behavior Monitoring Charts").

Ongoing Assessment of Therapy

The initiation of antipsychotic therapy is the beginning of an ongoing process of patient monitoring. The risk/benefit analysis must be continued throughout therapy. The goal of therapy should always be to use the least amount of medication that will result in the greatest possible benefit. If the goals of therapy are achieved, it might be appropriate to reduce the medication dosage or discontinue it altogether. If the goals are not achieved, then reevaluate therapy, consider a possible increase in dosage, or try an alternative therapy.

Chapter 16

DEFINING APPROPRIATE AND ACHIEVABLE OUTCOMES

Joanne Rader

After underlying needs have been identified and appropriate interventions chosen, it is time to define outcomes. Again, the task is to look at outcomes first from the resident's perspective. This means again weighing benefits and burdens. Here we will focus on outcomes related to psychoactive medications and physical restraints.

In relation to psychoactive medications, outcomes must be clearly defined. For example, the initiation of antipsychotic therapy is the beginning of an ongoing process of patient monitoring. Appropriate antipsychotic use can be encouraged by thoroughly considering the risks and benefits of therapy for a particular resident. The risk/benefit analysis must be continued throughout therapy.

The long-term goal related to the use of tie-on physical restraints is to eliminate their use in nursing homes and in the interim to consider their use temporary, always looking for the least restrictive form of restraint for the least amount of time. A companion goal is to maintain a reasonable margin of safety.

Expecting many behaviors to be completely eliminated is unrealistic. Success can mean that the difficult behaviors have been eliminated or have reached a level that is acceptable. Of course, the question is, acceptable to whom? If the underlying cause of yelling is pain, perhaps any amount of the pain would be intolerable to a resident, yet it may not be possible to completely eliminate it. If yelling indicates a reaction to environmental stress, caregivers must try to identify and eliminate the stress. If, however, the underlying cause of the yelling is related to the fear and distress of dementia, it may also be impossible to eliminate.

A variety of interventions may reduce the frequency and intensity of yelling related to dementia:

- Skillful reassurance
- Meaningful short activities
- Frequent, consistent staff contact
- Individual staff contact based on knowledge of the person

Decreased yelling may indicate reduced fear while providing an acceptable noise level for others in the environment.

Others' level of acceptance for any behavior will often vary from person to person and from day to day. That is why it is crucial to clearly identify what level can be accepted so that interventions are not left to the whims of individual staff members. The nurse supervisor can be most helpful by assuring that the acceptable level decided upon by the team (including the resident and family) represents the "highest practical level possible."

The concept of labeling behaviors as acceptable can be a double-edged sword. It is included so that the staff will not view complete elimination of behavioral symptoms as the only form of success and feel compelled to overtreat with approaches and medications. However, it is not meant to serve as an excuse to stop investigation. For example, after the resident is routinely medicated for arthritic pain, if he then yells only on the evening shift, you will still want to continue your investigation. His yelling may be related to a particular caregiver's approach or to fatigue.

In conclusion, the material in this book is designed to help readers develop new attitudes, approaches, and skills in caring for persons with difficult behavioral symptoms. The book has provided a guide through a thoughtful problem-solving process that includes taking on the roles of magician, detective, carpenter, and jester. It is hoped that some of the tedium and frustrations of coping with behavioral symptoms will be relieved when the staff rediscovers the magic of caring and the reason they are committed to this work. It is also hoped that this book will give the reader permission and encouragement to be creative and compassionate and develop a care system that treats others in the way that they themselves would wish to be treated.

The authors are cognizant of the many pushes and pulls in the current long-term care system and the health care system in general that make the magic of caring difficult to implement. But it has also been the authors' personal experience in changing practice related to the use of physical restraints that the biggest obstacles to change are not money or regulations or paperwork but our own biases, unwillingness to change, and fears. Therefore, providers, regulators, advocates, and consumers need to bravely and collectively hold hands and create new models and interventions based on the residents' perspective and wishes.

PART IV

APPENDICES

BEHAVIOR MONITORING CHARTS: INSTRUCTIONS FOR USE OF 24-HOUR BEHAVIOR MONITORING CHART

The 24-hour Behavior Monitoring Chart is an efficient tool for systematically recording behavioral symptoms. It can aid in identifying patterns of behavior (target behaviors) and possible causes and/or contributing factors. It also serves as documentation of changes in behavior resulting from interventions such as psychoactive medications. Monitoring should be initiated prior to starting any psychoactive medications or other interventions whenever possible.

To use the chart, first define the target behavior(s) to be observed and then customize the form for the resident whose behavior will be recorded. The specific steps are outlined below.

1. Define target behavior(s) to be observed
   a. Identify behavioral symptoms of concern. More than one symptom can be recorded on each form if needed.
   b. Develop a coding scheme to use in recording either (1) the presence or absence of the symptom or (2) the degree or severity of the symptom when it occurs. For example:
      0 = sleeping
      1 = restless
   or if you want additional information, it might be
      0 = no fall

1 = stumbled, lost balance but did not fall
2 − fell

If the behavior in question is calling out and you want to note the degree of disturbance exhibited, the coding might be:

0 = none, quiet
1 = occasional calling out (about 1/4 of the time)
2 = frequent calling out (around 1/2 of the time)
3 = continuous calling out (more than 3/4 of the time)

c. Carefully choose neutral rather than judgmental descriptive words. Accurately describe the behaviors observed and the continuum or range of behaviors. Discuss this with various staff members and shifts to be sure descriptions are clear and complete. Example: use "requests assistance 3–5 times per hour" rather than "demanding behavior."

2. Determine how often observations of the behaviors are to be recorded. Some behaviors may need recording only daily or once a shift. Others should be noted as often as every 2 hours. More frequent recording is probably not practical.

3. Customize the form:

a. Enter behavior to be coded and codes to be used in the space marked "Target Behavioral Symptoms" at the bottom of the form. This ensures that all staff using the form use the same notation.

Target Behavioral Symptoms: Calling out

---

0 = none, quiet
1 = occasional calling out
2 = frequent calling out
3 = continuous calling out

---

b. Enter observation intervals in spaces provided under "Time". The form is divided into 3 sections to correspond to shifts. Each section has a space where the nurse initials her documentation at the end of the shift. Each section is allotted 4 rows so that each 8-hour shift can be divided into 2-hour time intervals. Label the time intervals to correspond to shifts in your facility. You may wish to enter two code numbers into one time slot if a resident was engaging in more than one behavior during that time interval.

4. If desired, list interventions being evaluated in the space provided, or mark them on the grid. Psychoactive medications can be documented here.

5. Reviewing the observations and interventions:

   a. Review the sheet for the pattern of target behavior(s).

      Note:
      - frequency, time of day, shift
      - "Hi-liter" colors can accent the pattern of target behaviors

   b. Review the coding system to ensure that it still reflects the target behaviors.

      Note:
      - Avoid judgmental words: use calling for nurse 3–5 times per hour rather than "demanding behavior."
      - Avoid generalizations: use striking at staff with closed fist rather than "aggressive behavior."

   c. Review the possible underlying causes of the behavior. Are they reversible?

      Note:
      - hunger and/or thirst, discomfort related to being to cold or warm
      - medication interaction, dosage, or side effects
      - medical condition (UTI, constipation, pain)
      - environmental (noise, excess activity)
      - interpersonal (clash with staff, family, other residents)

   d. Review present interventions.

      Note:
      - Are they still useful?

- Are there new ones?
- Is problem solved?
- If applicable, record on monthly summary target symptoms response to psychoactive medications and any observed side effects.

6. When psychoactive medications are used, this sheet provides a concise way to assure that the necessary elements of documentation mandated in OBRA are present.

BEHAVIOR MONITORING CHART

MONTH/YR

Date / Time	1	2	3	4	5	6	7	8	9	10	11	12	13	14	15	16	17	18	19	20	21	22	23	24	25	26	27	28	29	30	31
Nurse's Initials																															
Nurse's Initials																															
Nurse's Initials																															

Target Behavioral Symptoms

0 —
1 —
2 —
3 —
4 —

Diagnosis:

Interventions:

A —
B —
C —
D —
E —

Date Initiated

NAME _____   MEDICATION _____   RECORD/ROOM # _____

Reverse side of behavior monitoring sheet looks like this:

INITIAL	SIGNATURE	TITLE	INITIAL	SIGNATURE	TITLE

Summary of target behavioral symptoms and response to interventions

_____

_____

_____

_____

_____

Monthly summary of psychoactive medication side effects (if applicable)

_____

_____

_____

_____

_____

BEHAVIOR MONITORING CHART (Example)   MONTH/YR September 1994

Time	1	2	3	4	5	6	7	8	9	10	11	12	13	14	15	16	17	18	19	20	21	22	23	24	25	26	27	28	29	30	31
2200–2400	2	2	2	0	0	0	2	2	0	0	0	0	0	0	0	0	0	0	0	0	0	0	0	0	0	0	0	0	0	0	0
2400–0200	0	2	0	2	0	0	0	2	2	0	0	0	0	0	0	0	0	0	0	0	0	0	0	0	0	2	0	0	0	0	0
0200–0400	2	0	2/4	0	2	2	0	2/4	0	0	2	2	0	0	0	0	0	2	0	0	0	2	0	0	0	0	0	0	0	0	0
0400–0600	0	0	4	0	0	2	0	0	0	0	0	0	2	2	2	0	0	0	0	0	0	0	0	0	0	0	0	0	2	0	2
Nurse's Initials																															
0600–0800	1	0	0	4	1	0	1	4	0	1	1	1	1	1	1	1	0	0	0	0	0	1	0	0	1	1	0	0	0	0	0
0800–1000	0	0	0	0	0	0	0	0	0	0	0	0	0	0	0	0	0	0	0	0	0	0	0	0	0	0	0	0	0	0	0
1000–1200	0	1	0	1	4	1	0	0	1	0	0	0	0	0	0	0	0	0	0	1	0	0	0	0	0	0	1	1	1	1	0
1200–1400	0	0	0	0	0	0	0	0	0	0	0	0	0	0	0	0	0	0	0	0	0	0	0	0	0	0	0	0	0	0	0
Nurse's Initials																															
1400–1600	0	0	0	0	0	0	0	0	0	0	0	0	0	0	0	0	0	0	0	0	0	0	0	0	0	0	0	0	0	0	0
1600–1800	1/4	0	0	1	0	0	0	1	4/1	1	0	0	1	0	0	0	0	0	0	0	0	0	0	0	0	0	0	0	0	0	0
1900–2000	4	4	0	4	0	4	0	0	0	4	4	4	4	4	0	0	0	4	0	1/4	0	0	0	0	4	0	0	0	1/4	0	0
2000–2400	0	3	0	4	0	0	4	3/4	0	0	0	0	0	4	4	4	0	0	0	0	4	4	0	0	0	0	4	0	0	0	0
Nurse's Initials																															

Diagnosis: Depression

Target Behavioral Symptoms

0 — No target symptoms
1 — Refusing to eat
2 — Insomnia
3 — Talks about suicide
4 — Sad and tearful

Interventions

A — Trazadone begun
B — Offered herbal tea when unable to sleep
C — Snacks offered when meals refused
D — Trazadone increased to 50 mg @ HS
E — Back rub offered when unable to sleep

	Date Initiated
A	8/3/94
B	9/1/94
C	9/1/94
D	9/10/94
E	9/25/94

Trazadone 25 mg @ HS

_____
NAME

_____
MEDICATION

_____
RECORD/ROOM #

EXAMPLE

INITIAL	SIGNATURE	TITLE	INITIAL	SIGNATURE	TITLE

Summary of target behavioral symptoms and response to interventions
9/30/94

S: "I seem to be sleeping better"

O: Trazadone 25 mg was initiated last month for depressive behavior
    (see target symptoms). Increased dose to 50 mg on 9/10/94. Marked
    decrease in target symptoms noted by end of this month.

A: Tolerating current dose well; improvement in symptoms. Tea and
    back rubs also seem effective for insomnia.

P: Continue with current medication, dose and comfort interventions.

Monthly summary of psychoactive medication side effects
9/30/94

Slight AM lethargy noted for 3 days following increased dose. None
noted now.

ASSESSMENT AND CARE PLANNING, THE KEY TO GOOD CARE: A GUIDE FOR NURSING HOME RESIDENTS AND THEIR FAMILIES

WHY DO YOU NEED TO KNOW ABOUT ASSESSMENT AND CARE PLANNING?

Every person in a nursing home has a right to good care, under the law. The law says the home must help people "attain or maintain" their highest level of well-being—physically, mentally and emotionally. To give good care staff must *assess* each resident and *plan care* to support each person's lifelong patterns and current interests, strengths, and needs. Resident and family involvement in care planning gives staff information they need to make sure residents get good care.

WHAT IS A RESIDENT ASSESSMENT?

Assessments gather information about how well residents can take care of themselves and when they need help in "functional abilities"—how well they can walk, talk, eat, dress, bathe, see, hear, communicate, understand, and remember. Staff also ask about residents' habits, activities, and relationships so that they can help residents live more comfortably and feel more at home.

The assessment helps staff look for what is causing a problem. For instance, poor balance could be caused by medications, sitting too much, weak muscles, poorly fitting shoes, a urinary infection, or an earache. Staff must know the cause in order to give treatment.

WHAT IS A PLAN OR CARE?

A plan of care is a strategy for how the staff will help a resident. It says what each staff person will do and when it will happen (for instance, the nursing assistant will help Mrs. Jones walk to each meal to build her strength). Care plans must be reviewed regularly to make sure they work and must be revised as needed. For care plans to work, residents must feel they meet their needs and must be comfortable with them. Care plans can address any medical or non-medical problem (example: incompatibility with a roommate).

WHAT IS A CARE PLANNING CONFERENCE?

Care planning meetings must occur every 3 months and whenever there is a big change in a resident's physical or mental health that might require a change in care. The care plan must be done within 7 days after an assessment. Assessments must be done within 14 days of admission and at least once a year, with reviews every 3 months and when a resident's condition changes.

WHAT SHOULD YOU TALK ABOUT
AT THE MEETING?

Talk about what you need, how you feel; ask questions about care and the daily routine, about food, activities, interests, staff, personal care, medications, how well you get around. Staff must talk to you about treatment decisions, such as medications and restraints and can only do what you agree to. You may have to be persistent about your concerns and choices. For help with problems, contact your local "ombudsman," advocacy group, or others listed on the next page.

HOW RESIDENTS AND THEIR FAMILIES CAN PARTICIPATE IN CARE PLANNING

Residents have the right to make choices about care, services, daily schedule, and life in the facility and to be involved in the care planning meeting. Participating is the only way to be heard.

Before the meeting:

- Tell staff how you feel, your concerns, what help you need or questions you have; plan your agenda of questions, problems, and goals for yourself and your care.
- Know, or ask your doctor or the staff, about your condition, care and treatment.
- Ask staff to hold the meeting when your family can come, if you want them there.

During the meeting:

- Discuss options for treatment and for meeting your needs and preferences. Ask questions if you need terms or procedures explained to you.
- Be sure you understand and agree with the care plan and feel it meets your needs. Ask for a copy of your care plan; ask with whom to talk if you need changes in it.

After the meeting:

- See how your care plan is followed; talk with nurse aides, other staff, or the doctor about it.

Families:

- Support your relative's agenda, choices, and participation in the meeting.

- Even if your relative has dementia, involve her/him in care planning as much as possible. Always assume that s/he may understand and communicate at some level. Help the staff find ways to communicate with and work with your relative.
- Help watch how the care plan is working and talk with staff if questions arise.

A Good Care Plan Should:

- be specific, individualized and written in common language that everyone can understand
- reflect residents' concerns and support residents' well-being, functioning and rights; not label residents' choices or needs as "problem behaviors"
- use a multidisciplinary team approach and use outside referrals as needed
- be reevaluated and revised routinely. Watch for care plans that never change.

If you need help, contact National Citizen's Coalition for Nursing Home Reform, 1224 "M" Street, N. W., Suite 301, (202) 393-2018.

Used with permission from the National Citizen's Coalition for Nursing Home Reform, July 1992.

GUIDELINES FOR MANAGING BEHAVIORAL EMERGENCIES IN THE NURSING HOME SETTING

DEFINITION

A behavioral emergency occurs when there is a sudden, generally unexpected change or escalation in the behavior of a resident that is perceived to pose a serious threat to the safety of the resident or others and appears to demand immediate action.

On occasion, nursing home staff are confronted with behavioral emergencies in which the health and safety of a resident or others is being eminently threatened. Available interdisciplinary staff should determine whether a particular behavior constitutes an emergency, as different observers may view the behavior differently, depending on their past experience, facility and regulatory rules, and other factors (Sternberg & Whelihan, 1991). Behavioral emergencies are often the result of some unidentified or untreated need or problem. Most behaviors can be defused and managed if the warning signs are identified and early intervention done to prevent or slow escalation. Infrequently some incidents occur quickly and without warning. Therefore, it is helpful to have a plan in place to handle situations in ways that provide for the safety and best interest of all involved. The following guidelines are designed to help you with this planning.

Stemberg, J., & Whelihan, W. (1991). Assessment of disruptive behavior in the nursing home: Stories and strategies. *Rhode Island Medical Journal, 74*, 81–95 and others.

EXAMPLES OF POSSIBLE BEHAVIORAL EMERGENCIES

1. Significant physical aggression unresponsive to staff interventions such as redirection, diversion
2. Significant acts of sexual aggression unresponsive to staff interventions
3. Hiding things which could be used as weapons (e.g., glassware, silverware)
4. Suicidal threats or gestures (e.g., hiding and hoarding medications)

PRIORITIES

1. Insuring the safety of the resident and others
2. A swift assessment of the cause underlying the behavioral symptom
3. Determining the most appropriate and realistic 24-hour treatment plan
4. Initiating changes in the resident's care plan

PROCEDURE

The following steps are suggested to address these priorities:

1. Secure the situation.
2. Assess the problem.
3. Develop a plan for completion of shift.
4. Modify existing care plan.

STEP 1—SECURE THE SITUATION

The staff must determine what the safety issues are and what is required to immediately create a safer environment for the resident and others

a. Immediately designate an emergency coordinator. It is critical that one individual in the facility be in charge of the situation. Initially, if there is violence being committed, the first person on the scene assumes this role until they are relieved of that responsibility. The coordinator may be the resident care manager, director of nursing services, social worker, administrator, or a variety of other staff members. If there is someone on staff with experience in handling behavioral emergencies and they are available, this would be a logical person to assume this role. Your facility may wish to designate someone to routinely serve in this role or have it change depending on the resident and type of behavioral emergency. This person serves as the contact person for others, such as the family, physician, mental health worker, and police.

All actions, information, and decisions are routed through the coordinator. The coordinator may delegate tasks but will need to be aware of what others are doing and saying.

If the determination is made that significant violence is occurring or about to occur, the coordinator should call 911 and ask for police assistance.

b. Isolate the Individual. A way to have that individual separate from the rest of the population may need to be created. This can be done by temporarily moving a roommate or using an office or therapy room.

c. Assess the environment for safety risks and ways to modify the environment to reduce those risks. For example, look to see if there are objects in the environment that can be used as weapons and remove them. Check the resident to see if he or she has any concealed weapons.

d. If needed, get additional help to provide immediate one-to-one monitoring, to insure safety. It is useful to engage the person who in the past has worked best with the resident and has his/her trust if they are readily available.

STEP 2—ASSESS THE PROBLEM

When there is a sudden behavioral change, it is crucial that staff assume that this behavior is a symptom of some unidentified or untreated underlying cause and that they begin action to determine what that cause is. This includes

a. looking at the "ABCs" of the immediate situation—what were the **antecedents** (what occurred just prior to the behavior), what was **behavior**, and what were the **consequences** (what occurred right after the behavior)—for possible causes or things that may have escalated the situation.

Basically staff should do a head-to-toe assessment even if it can only be done by looking at the individual. You will be looking for such things as causes for delirium, possible strokes, pain, social and environmental changes or losses, etc. It is important for the staff to determine if individual has dementia, if the behavior was a catastrophic reaction precipitated by staff approaches or environmental stressors.

b. gathering as much data as possible about current physical status, such as vital signs, blood sugar levels, voiding, or signs of injury, unless to do so poses too much risk or will escalate the situation.

c. reviewing the chart, including current medications, behavioral flow sheets (if available), presence of any acute illnesses, medical and psychiatric history, any recent losses or environmental changes, and any other information deemed pertinent.

STEP 3—DEVELOP PLAN FOR COMPLETION OF SHIFT

The coordinator should be developing a plan to get through the shift. He or she completes or delegates the following tasks.

a. Call a family member to inform them of the behavior change. If the family member or significant other is an active part of the treatment team, they need to be notified immediately and given the opportunity to participate in decision making. It is important to ask if this current behavior has occurred in the

past, and if so, what the underlying cause and treatment
were.

b. RN or LPN to contact the physician and

1. describe the behavior in specific terms, including the onset, course, all data in step 2, and immediate interventions
done in step 1

2. request any lab work or tests that you think are needed

3. ask what he/she would recommend

c. Contact the identified mental health resource person. Every
facility should have a mental health resource person identified that they can call in an emergency. This may be someone
on staff, an outside consultant, or someone from the crisis
service of the local community mental health program.
Facility Mental Health Resource Person
Name: _____
Phone: _____

1. Describe the behavior in specific terms, including onset,
course, all data in step 2, and interventions done in step 1.

2. Request consultation regarding possible interventions.
This may be done by phone or on site, depending on your
available local resources.

d. At this point, the coordinator develops a plan for the rest of
the shift. This may include such interventions as one-to-one
supervision, isolation from other residents, medication,
physical restraint, and transfer to a more secure environment.

e. Complete documentation: Document the behavioral symptom. This may include a narrative note and/or a behavior
flow sheet and writing a summary of the incident and interventions in the chart.

STEP 4—MODIFY EXISTING CARE PLAN

It is critical for the health team to determine what the appropriate
plan of care would be for the rest of the day and the next few days.
Often after a frightening incident, staff and facilities feel the only

solution is to remove the resident from the facility. However, this may not be the best course of action for the resident and, with consultation and planning, often another plan of care can be devised that addresses the safety of others in the facility. To develop this plan it is important to mobilize the existing mental health resources and involve professionals that are familiar with dealing with a mental health crisis. This may take 1–2 days to complete.

a. Mobilize the interdisciplinary treatment team to address on-going care needs and how to prevent reoccurrences of the behavioral emergencies. This may include contacting
   1. Senior and Disabled Services Division (SDSD) case worker if resident is Medicaid client (local office phone # _____)
   2. local mental health office to discuss need for an annual resident review (ARR) under Preadmission screening and Annual Resident Review (PASARR) process (local office phone # _____)
   3. your facility mental health consultant if other than PASAAR
   4. master of social work (MSW) consultant if the facility social worker is not an MSW
   5. family
   6. physician
   7. psychiatrist if the resident has or is being seen by one
   8. other state mental health resources
   Include the resident in decision making at whatever level appears appropriate and possible, given their crisis situation.
b. Develop a plan to maintain stabilization for 72 hours.
c. Debrief with the staff involved to
   1. allow them to express and let go of any fears or feelings related to the behavior
   2. see if they can at this point identify any additional factors that might have caused or precipitated the behavior

3. identify what they have learned that might be helpful in the future with this client and others.

SUMMARY CHECKLIST FOR MANAGING BEHAVIORAL EMERGENCIES IN THE NURSING HOME SETTING

Step 1—Secure the Situation

- Immediately designate an emergency coordinator
- Isolate the individual
- Assess the environment for safety risks
- If needed, get additional help

Step 2—Assess the Problem

- Looking at the "ABC's" of the immediate situation
- Gather as much data as possible
- Review the chart

Step 3—Develop a Plan for Completion of Shift

- Call a family member.
- RN or LPN to contact the physician.
- Contact an identified mental health resource person if unable to manage situation.
- Develop a plan for the rest of the shift.
- Complete documentation.

Step 4—Modify Existing Care Plan

- Mobilize the interdisciplinary treatment team.
- Develop a plan to maintain stabilization for 72 hours.
- Debrief staff

THE FREEDOM TO BE RESTRAINT-FREE: INFORMATION ABOUT PHYSICAL RESTRAINTS FOR NURSING HOME RESIDENTS, FAMILIES, AND FRIENDS

FREEDOM TO CHOOSE

There have been some exciting changes in the philosophy and practice of delivering care to nursing home residents. One especially positive development, supported by federal mandate, is a renewed emphasis on promoting dignity by increasing freedom of choice.

As a result of this new emphasis, more and more nursing homes are shifting to individualized rehabilitative approaches to care. A rehabilitative approach means that each resident is provided help in attaining or maintaining his or her highest level of independence and functional capacity, with care and care routines centered on the particular needs of each person. Such individualized care is based on full respect for the resident as an adult with fundamental rights, including freedom of choice and movement.

This philosophy of care has resulted in a dramatic change in thinking about the use of physical restraints. This pamphlet

This material was developed as part of the Robert Wood Johnson Foundation Grant #17311 answers some questions you might have about the use of physical restraints.

PHYSICAL RESTRAINTS

1. What is a physical restraint?

The most common examples are vests or belts that tie the resident to a bed or chair, "geriatric" chairs with lapboards, or full bedrails that are intended to prevent standing and independent transfer.

A physical restraint is any device that restricts freedom of movement. Of concern are devices attached or adjacent to the body that limit movement, do not reflect resident choice, and are not under resident control.

2. Why are restraints used and how effective are they?

In the last few years it has become clear that the benefits of restraints were greatly overestimated, while the tremendous physical, social, and psychological burden they created for the individual was not considered. Restraints were used in an attempt to prevent falls or unattended "wandering," but their effectiveness had never been tested. There is now evidence that many restraints are unsafe: vest and waist restraints have caused a number of deaths, and findings from recent studies suggest that restraints may actually increase the risk of injury when a fall occurs.

Tying residents to chairs or beds often worsens physical and mental disabilities because restraints limit the ability to perform physical and mental exercise. Reduced activity imposed by restraints leads to increased weakness and confusion that often results in more falls and more fall-related injuries. Full bedrails often add to the risk of injury from falling as residents frequently attempt to climb over them.

We have learned that we can develop reasonable safety plans without severely restricting residents' mobility. Using individualized approaches based on comprehensive assessments, many facilities have become "restraint-free."

Occasionally, short-term use of a restraint may be required in an emergency. According to 1992 federal guidelines, if there are medical symptoms which are life threatening, a restraint may be used temporarily to facilitate lifesaving treatment if there is evidence that the resident or legal representative approves of the treatment. Restraints may also be used if the resident's behavior is posing an immediate threat to the safety of others.

3. What changes can you expect because of this reduction in the use of physical restraints?

Nursing home staff use creative alternatives to restraints as they try to support the dignity of the resident while promoting mobility and safety. For some residents, this means lowering beds closer to the floor, providing comfortable seating systems, or providing small alarms that alert the staff when the resident needs assistance. You may observe residents who appear somewhat unsteady when walking, but walking strengthens their bones and muscles. Restraint reduction has focused attention on environmental contributions to mobility and safety. So you may also observe changes in the environment, or be asked to participate in evaluation of equipment or training methods designed to increase safe mobility.

Because physical and mental difficulties are pervasive among nursing home residents, there will continue to be residents who fall. Facilities that have eliminated restraints report that although the number of falls may stay the same or even increase, there has been no corresponding increase in injuries related to falls. These facilities also report dramatic decreases in agitated behavior and yelling and a generally more caring, compassionate environment for residents, family, and staff.

4. What role can family and friends play?

Relatives and friends play a vital role in helping the nursing home staff individualize care by providing information about the resident's life experiences and customary daily routine. Relatives can also support the staff's efforts to reduce or eliminate restraint use.

Some specific ways families and friends can be of assistance include

- bringing in familiar objects, such as favorite chairs or decorative items for the bedroom
- creating individualized activity kits such as purses or tool boxes that have meaning for the resident
- helping the residents maintain their ability to walk by walking with them
- sharing observations and concerns with the staff. You may be able to help the staff identify the causes and appropriate responses to behavioral symptoms you have dealt with in the past

These helpful approaches vary with the physical and mental skills of the individual resident, and families are encouraged to work with staff to assure that plans are coordinated and appropriate. The change in attitude and practice has generally been welcomed by facilities, staff, residents, and families once they become aware of the facts about restraints.

Negative Consequences of Restraint Use You Need to Know About

- Withdrawal, humiliation, depression, regressive behavior, resistance, anger, agitation
- Complications of restricted mobility, including circulatory obstruction, edema or swelling, pressure ulcers, muscle wasting, joint contractures, osteoporosis, respiratory problems, infection, increased incontinence, and a drop in blood pressure when standing
- Increased confusion, decreased appetite, dehydration.
- Changes in body chemistry due to responses to stress
- Injuries and deaths related to restraint use

For additional information contact

Alzheimer's Association
919 North Michigan Avenue, Suite 1000
Chicago, IL 60611-1676
(312) 335-8700

American Association of Homes for the Aging
901 E Street NW, Suite 500
Washington, DC 20004-2037
(202) 783-2242

American Health Care Association
1201 L Street NW
Washington, DC 20005
(202) 842-4444

National Citizens' Coalition for Nursing Home Reform
1224 M Street, NW, Suite 301
Washington, DC 20005-5183
(202) 393-2018

PSYCHOACTIVE MEDICATION INFORMATION SHEETS

GENERAL NOTE RELATED TO PSYCHOACTIVE MEDICATION INFORMATION SHEETS

These sheets contain simplified, condensed information and are meant to be used as general guides only. The dosages listed are maximum daily doses for individuals who have organic mental syndrome or who are elderly. Readers are advised to consult more detailed sources of information if they have questions about a particular medication and dosage.

Individuals, particularly the elderly, differ in the amount of drug needed for treatment without side effects. Some patients may have side effects at very low doses, while others may benefit from doses higher than the maximum. If high doses are used, ask the following questions:

- Were lower doses tried?
- Were they ineffective?
- Were there no side effects?

If the lower dose was ineffective and there were no side effects, then a higher dose may be used.

ANTIPSYCHOTIC MEDICATION INFORMATION SHEET

Diagnoses Pertinent to Antipsychotic Use

1. Schizophrenia
2. Schizoaffective disorder
3. Delusional disorder
4. Psychotic mood disorder (including mania and depression with psychotic features)
5. Acute psychotic episodes
6. Brief reactive psychosis
7. Schizophreniform disorder
8. Atypical psychosis
9. Tourette's disorder
10. Huntington's disease
11. Organic mental syndromes (including dementia) with associated psychotic and/or agitated state defined by specific, quantitative behaviors, objectively documented as representing a danger to the resident and others (including staff).

Examples of Symptoms for Treatment Related to Organic Mental Syndrome:

1. Continuous yelling, crying out, screaming, or pacing if these specific behaviors cause an impairment in functional capacity
2. Psychotic symptoms such as hallucinations, paranoia, or delusions if these behaviors cause an impairment in functional capacity.

Examples of target symptoms

- Biting staff on a daily basis
- Scratching roommate at least once a week
- Refusing any type of care continuously on evening shift

Antipsychotics should *not* be used for individual symptoms such as wandering, poor self-care, restlessness, impaired memory, anxiety, depression, insomnia, unsociability, indifference to surroundings, fidgeting, nervousness, uncooperativeness, unspecified agitation.

When using antipsychotic drugs, testing for abnormal involuntary movements is suggested upon initiation of the drug and every 6 months. Abnormal Involuntary Movement Scale (AIMS) and Dyskinesia Identification System Condensed User Scale (DISCUS) are two commonly used tools.

Commonly Used Antipsychotics

Generic	Brand	Maximum Daily Dose for Organic Mental Syndrome
Thioridazine	Mellaril	75 mg
Perphenazine	Trilafon	8 mg
Trifluoperazine	Stelazine	8 mg
Thiothixene	Navane	7 mg
Haloperidol	Haldol	4 mg
Loxapine	Loxitane	10 mg

ANTIPSYCHOTIC SIDE EFFECT PROFILE

Side Effects of Antipsychotics:

1. Drowsiness and sedation
2. Extrapyramidal effects (EPS): dystonias (muscle spasms of eye, neck, and back), akathisia (motor restlessness, esp. in elderly female), parkinsonism (stiffness and rigidity, esp. in elderly female), akinesia (markedly decreased body activity)
3. Tardive dyskinesia (TD): involuntary, repetitive, purposeless movements involving the eyes, face, mouth, tongue, trunk, and limbs
4. Cardiovascular effects: peripheral vasodilatation, orthostatic hypotension, tachycardia, ECG changes, arrhythmia

5. Anticholinergic effects: decreased gastric, bronchial, and salivary secretions (causing symptoms such as dry mouth, blurred vision, and nasal congestion); reduced spasms of smooth muscle in the bladder, bronchi, and intestine (causing symptoms such as constipation, delayed micturition reflex or urinary retention)
6. Endocrine effects: inhibition of ejaculation, weight gain
7. Skin reactions: photosensitivity, rashes
8. Ocular effects: lenticular pigmentation, pigmentary retinopathy

---

Warning: Residents should be *tapered off slowly* when medication is discontinued.

Commonly Used Antipsychotics and Their Side Effect Profile

Generic	Brand	Maximum Daily Dose for Organic Mental Syndrome	Sedation	Extrapyramidal Effects	Anticholinergic Effects	Cardiovascular Effects
Thioridazine	Mellaril	75 mg	high	low	high	high
Perphenazine	Trilafon	8 mg	low	high	low	low
Trifluoperazine	Stelazine	8 mg	low	high	low	low
Thiothixene	Navane	7 mg	low	high	low	low
Haloperidol	Haldol	4 mg	low	very high	low	low
Loxapine	Loxitane	10 mg	low	very high	low	low

Adverse reactions such as dystonic reactions warrant discontinuation of the antipsychotic agent. Specific examples include

- oculogyric crisis: fixed upward gaze
- torticollis: neck twisting
- opisthotonos: arching of back
- trismus: clenched jaw
- neuroleptic malignant syndrome (NMS): hypothermia, skeletal muscle rigidity, autonomic nervous system dysfunction (tachycardia, increased or decreased blood pressure)

- others: spasm of muscle group resulting in facial grimaces, exaggerated posturing of head or jaw, difficulty in speech, swallowing, breathing

ANTIDEPRESSANT MEDICATION INFORMATION SHEET

Diagnoses Pertinent to Antidepressant Use

In general mood disorders, including

1. major depression, single episode or recurrent, mild, moderate, severe, with or without psychotic features or unspecified
2. dysthymia
3. depressive disorder not otherwise specified
4. bipolar disorder, mixed, depressed
5. cyclothymia
6. bipolar disorder not otherwise specified

Antidepressants may also be useful in treating some types of insomnia and as an adjunct in pain management. Antidepressants are generally not helpful in treating situational or secondary depression. That is why a thorough assessment is important.

Examples of Symptoms for Treatment Related to Major Depression

1. Depressed mood most of the day, nearly every day (observed or subjective)
2. Diminished pleasure or interest in activities most of the day, nearly every day
3. Significant weight loss or gain (> or <5% of body weight in a month)
4. Insomnia or hypersomnia nearly every night
5. Psychomotor agitation or retardation (observed by others)

6. Fatigue or loss of energy nearly every day
7. Feeling worthless, helpless, or hopeless
8. Inappropriate or excessive feelings of guilt
9. Decreased ability to think or concentrate or indecisiveness nearly every day
10. Recurrent thoughts of death, suicidal ideations with or without a plan
11. Suicide attempt
12. Delusions or hallucinations whose content is consistent with typical depressive themes of personal inadequacy (e.g., guilt, disease, death, nihilism, or deserved punishment).
13. Same as above but does not involve typical depressive themes. Delusions include persecutory, thought insertion/broadcasting, and delusions of control.

Commonly Used Antidepressants

Generic	Brand	Maximum Daily Dose Range
Desipramine	Norpramin	25–100 mg
Doxepin	Sinequan	25–75 mg
Fluoxetin	Prozac	20 mg
Nortriptyline	Pamelor	10–75 mg
Protriptyline	Vivactil	5–30 mg
Trazadone	Desyrel	25–200 mg

ANTIDEPRESSANT SIDE EFFECT PROFILE

Common Side Effects of Antidepressants

1. Anticholinergic effects: decreased gastric, bronchial, and salivary secretions (such as dry mouth, blurred vision, and nasal congestion); reduced spasms of smooth muscle in the bladder, bronchi, and intestine (such as constipation, delayed micturition reflex, or urinary retention)
2. CNS effects: drowsiness, sedation, insomnia, excitement, confusion, headache, lower seizure threshold

3. Cardiovascular effects: orthostatic hypotension, dizziness, tachycardia, ECG changes, cardiac arrhythmia
4. GI distress: nausea
5. Others: rash, fatigue, weight gain, sexual disturbances, and epileptic seizures; in addition, some antidepressants may have extrapyramidal side effects (EPS).

> **Warning:** Residents should be *tapered off slowly* when medication is discontinued.

Commonly Used Antidepressants and Their Side Effects Profile

Generic	Brand	Maximum Daily Dose Range	Anticholinergic Potency	Sedation	Seizures	Orthostasis	Arhythmias
Desipramine	Norpramin	25–50 mg	++	++	++	+++	+++
Doxepin	Sinequan	25–75 mg	+++	++++	+++	++	++
Fluoxetin	Prozac	20 mg	+	++	−	+	−
Nortriptyline	Pamelor	10–75 mg	+++	+++	++	+	+++
Protriptyline	Vivactil	5–30 mg	+++	+	++	++	++++
Trazadone	Desyrel	25–200 mg	−	+++	++	+++	+

Avoid in older adults because of high level of side effects; use only in specified conditions:

Generic	Brand	Maximum Daily Dose Range	Anticholinergic Potency	Sedation	Seizures	Orthostasis	Arhythmias
Amitriptyline	Elavil	25–100 mg	++++	++++	+++	+++	++++
Amoxapine	Ascendin	50–100 mg	+++	++	+++	+	++
Imipramine	Tofranil	25–100 mg	+++	+++	+++	++++	++++

ANXIOLYTIC (ANTIANXIETY) MEDICATION INFORMATION SHEET

Diagnoses Pertinent to Antianxiety Use

1. Generalized anxiety disorder
2. Panic disorder

3. Agoraphobia
4. Simple phobia
5. Posttraumatic disorder
6. Depression with symptoms of anxiety, anxiety disorder not otherwise specifiying
7. Organic mental syndrome including dementia with an associated agitated state defined by specific, quantitative behaviors, objectively documented as representing a danger to the resident or others.

Examples of Symptoms of Treatment

Examples related to *generalized anxiety disorder may include* unrealistic excessive worry about two or more life circumstances, trembling, twitching, feeling shaky, muscle tension, aches, soreness, restlessness, feeling easily fatigued, shortness of breath, smothering sensation, palpitations, tachycardia, sweating, cold clammy hands, dry mouth, dizziness, flushes or chills, feeling "keyed up" or "on edge," exaggerated startle response, difficulty concentrating, mind "going blank," trouble falling or staying asleep, irritability.

Examples related to *organic mental syndrome may include* slapping staff on all shifts on a daily basis, biting self daily leaving open wounds, screaming all afternoon causing resident to be short of breath and diaphoretic, pushing other residents down whenever they come into his/her space.

Most anxiolytic medications used are benzodiazepines (BZDs).

Commonly Used Short-Acting Anxiolytics

Generic	Brand	Maximum Daily Dose for Elderly
Alprazolam	Xanax	0.75 mg
Lorazepam	Ativan	2 mg
Oxazepam	Serax	30 mg
Buspirone*	BuSpar	30 mg

*Not BZD.

ANXIOLYTIC (ANTIANXIETY) SIDE EFFECT PROFILE

Side Effects of Benzodiazepine (BZD) Anxiolytics

1. CNS depression: extensions of the sedative effect such as fatigue, drowsiness, nystagmus, muscle weakness, hangover, and dysarthria (poorly articulated speech), esp. in elderly
2. Paradoxical agitation: insomnia, hallucinations, nightmares, hostility, violent behaviors, esp. in elderly
3. Confusion and disorientation, esp. in elderly
4. Amnesia (loss of memory)

> **Warning:** Residents should be *tapered off slowly* when medication is discontinued as these drugs are habit-forming, and withdrawal symptoms may occur.

Drugs that should *not* be used for the treatment of anxiety disorders include Benadryl, Atarax, and Vistaril.

In addition, the long-acting benzodiazepine (BZD) such as

chlordiazepoxide (Librium)
clorazepate (Tranxene)
prazepam (Centrax)
diazepam (Valium)
clonazepam (Klonopin)

should *not* be used with residents over the age of 65 unless an attempt with shorter-acting drugs has failed.

Commonly Used Short-Acting Anxiolytics

Generic	Brand	Maximum Daily Dose for Elderly	Drug Half-Life
Alprazolam	Xanax	0.75 mg	12–15 hours
Lorazepam	Ativan	2 mg	10–16 hours
Oxazepam	Serax	30 mg	5–20 hours
Buspirone*	BuSpar	30 mg	2–11 hours

*Not BZD.

SEDATIVE/HYPNOTIC INFORMATION SHEET

Insomnia is defined as difficulty in falling or staying asleep and/or not feeling refreshed upon awakening in the morning. Before obtaining an order for a sedative/hypnotic, an assessment should be done on the etiology of insomnia.

Insomnia can arise from several underlying causes. Insomnia can be classified in six general areas:

1. Situational insomnia (e.g., job stress, hospitalization, travel)
2. Medical insomnia (e.g., pain, respiratory problems, GI problems)
3. Psychiatric insomnia (e.g., schizophrenia, depression, mania, neurosis)
4. Drug intake insomnia (e.g., alcohol, caffeine, sympathomimetics)
5. Drug withdrawal insomnia (e.g., alcohol, anxiolytics, hypnotics, REM-suppressant drugs)
6. Primary or idiopathic insomnia

Diagnosis and effective treatment of the cause can usually eliminate the need for using hypnotic drugs. Remember these are habit-forming drugs!

Examples of Symptoms for Treatment Related to Primary or Idiopathic Insomnia

1. Difficulty in initiating and maintaining sleep at least three times a week for 1 month
2. Feeling unrested in the morning at least three times a week for 1 month.
3. Feeling unrested in the morning at least three times a week for 1 month, daytime.
4. Fatigue, irritability, impaired daytime functioning

Most sedative hypnotics used are benzodiazepines (BZDs).

Commonly Used Hypnotics

Generic	Brand	Maximum Daily Dose for Elderly
Temazepam	Restoril	15 mg
Triazolam	Halcion	0.125 mg
Zolpidem*	Ambien	5 mg

*Not BZD.

SEDATIVE/HYPNOTIC AGENTS SIDE EFFECT PROFILE

Side Effects of Benzodiazepine (BZDs)

1. CNS depression: extensions of the sedative effect such as fatigue, drowsiness, nystagmus, muscle weakness
2. Paradoxical agitation: insomnia, hallucinations, nightmares, hostility, violent behaviors, esp. in elderly
3. Confusion and disorientation, esp. in elderly
4. Amnesia (loss of memory)

> **Warning:** These drugs are habit-forming. Residents should be tapered off slowly.

Hypnotics should not be given 7 nights a week because people can develop a tolerance to these medications and require higher doses. Try giving sedative/hypnotics only 4 or 5 nights out of 7.

Commonly Used Hypnotics

Generic	Brand	Maximum Daily Dose for Elderly	Drug Half-Life
Temazepam	Restoril	15 mg	12.4 hours
Triazolam	Halcion	0.125 mg	2.5 hours
Zolpidem*	Ambien	5 mg	2.5 hours

*Not BZD.

RESOURCE LIST

This list includes products that various facilities and individuals have reported as useful. The list is not to be considered an endorsement for any products, and prior to purchasing a product it is advised that you obtain more information from the company or other providers to assure that the product is appropriate for the intended use.

PRINTED MATERIALS

Aging in the Designed Environment, M. Christenson, Hawthorne Press, 10 Alice Street, Binghamton, NY 13904-1580; 1990. This book provides detailed information on how to adapt the physical environment to compensate for sensory changes common to aging, enhance independence in the home and redesign long-term care facilities. An excellent resource for modifying the environment. $19.95.

An Ombudsman Guide to Effective Advocacy Regarding the Inappropriate Use of Chemical and Physical Restraint, National Citizens' Coalition for Nursing Home Reform (NCCNHR), 1224 "M" St., NW, Suite 301, Washington, DC 20005-5183. NCCNHR is offering these papers by Sarah Burger developed for the National Center for State Long Term Care Ombudsman Resources, funded by the Administration on Aging. They include a resource paper ($10) and trainer's guide ($5). The resource paper and trainer's guide can be purchased together for $13.75. Add 10% for postage and handling.

Avoiding Physical Restraint Use: New Standards of Care. A guide for residents, families, and friends. Sarah Burger, National Coalition for Nursing Home Reform, 1224 "M" Street, NW, #301, Washington, DC 20005, (202)393-2018. This booklet is helpful for families. $6.50 each; discount for five or more. Call for information.

Avoiding Drugs Used as Chemical Restraints: New Standards of Care. A guide for residents, families, friends, and caregivers. Sarah Burger, National Coalition for Nursing Home Refort, 1224 "M" Street, NW, #301, Washington, DC 20005-5183, (202)393-2018. Clear and concise, the guide explains the resident's right to be treated with dignity and respect and to have his or her individual needs met without unnecessary drugs. $6.50 each; discount for five or more. Call for information.

Care of the Alzheimer's Patient: A Manual for Nursing Home Staff, L. Gwyther, Alzheimer's Disease and Related Disorders Association (ADRDA), 1985. Obtain a copy by calling your local chapter or the national ADRDA (312)335-8700. An excellent resource. Cost is approximately $6–8.

Designing for Dementia: Planning Environments for the Elderly and the Confused, M. P. Calkins. National Health Publishing, 428 E. Preston St., Baltimore, MD 21202, (800)446-2221; 1988. This book is an excellent source of ideas on how to arrange, design, and structure the physical environment to allow persons with dementia to function better. $38.50 (plus $7 shipping).

Doing Things, J. M. Zgola, Johns Hopkins University Press, Hampton Station, Baltimore, MD 21211, (401)516-6956; 1987. This book offers a guide to programming activities for persons with Alzheimer's disease and related disorders. $10.95; $28.00 hardcover (plus $2 shipping).

For Those Who Take Care: An Alzheimer's Disease Training Program for Nursing Assistants, B. J. Helm, and D. R. Wekstein, Alzheimer's Disease Research Center, Dept. ADC, PO Box 8250, Silver Spring, MD 20907-8250. 45 slides, 182-p. manual and handouts. $50/set.

Holding On To Home: Designing Environments for People with Dementia, U. Cohen, and G. D. Weisman, The John Hopkins University

Press, Hampden Station, Baltimore, MD 21211. This book discusses the relationship between the physical environment, behavior and persons with dementia. It describes a variety of settings and would be particularly useful when considering building or remodeling a facility. $45 plus $3 shipping and handling.

Managing Behavior Problems in Nursing Home Residents: A Manual for Nursing Home Staff, J. A. Taylor, and W. A. Ray, Vanderbilt University School of Medicine, Department of Preventive Medicine, A1124 Medical Center N, Nashville, TN 37232, (615)322-2017; 1990. Continuing Education for Nursing Homes in Tennessee project. This is a good guide for staff on how to decrease inappropriate use of psychoactive medications and develop alternative ways to manage behavioral symptoms. $10. A free reprint *Managing Behavior Problems in Nursing Home Residents* is also available.

Optimum Care of the Nursing Home Resident with Alzheimer's Disease: "Giving a Little Extra", E. L. Ballard, and L. P. Gwyther, The Duke Family Support Program, P.O. Box 3600, Duke University Medical Center, Durham, NC 27710, (919)660-7510; 1991. Manual $10 (postage and handling included).

Reducing Inappropriate Restraint Use, NCCNHR, 1224 "M" St., NW, Suite 301, Washington, DC 20005-5183. Has resource packets on restraints, including materials from the December 4, 1989, Senate Special Committee on Aging symposium, "Untie the Elderly," and additional information on physical and chemical restraints and ways nursing homes are eliminating them. Packet "A" has information on why we need to decrease restraints. Packet "B" gives information on how to do it. $15/each (add 10% for postage and handling).

Reducing Restraints: Individualized Approaches to Behavior, N. E. Strumpf, J. Wagner, L. K. Evans, J. E. Patterson, Geriatric Resource and Training Center, 3501 Masons Hill Road, Suite 501-B, Huntingdon Valley, PA 19006, (215)657-9990; 1992. 10-session education program focuses on myths, effects, and legal and ethical issues regarding restraints and describes a method for making sense of behaviors that often lead to physical restraints.

Major emphasis is given to systematic ways to intervene with various behaviors. An important component focuses on the process of initiating and maintaining change. $75 (plus $3 shipping).

Toward a Restraint-Free Environment: Reducing the use of physical restraints in long-term care and acute care settings, Ed. J. V. Braun and S. Lopson, Health Profession Press, P.O. Box 10624, Baltimore, MD 21285-0624, (410)337-9585. This book provides step-by-step guidance and many helpful tools for restraint reduction. $28.00 (add 10% shipping and handling); if prepaid, no shipping and handling is charged.

Understanding Difficult Behaviors: Some Practical Suggestions for Coping with Alzheimer's Disease and Related Illnesses, A. Robinson, B. Spencer, L. White, The Alzheimer's Program, 5401 McAuley Dr., P.O. Box 994, Ann Arbor, MI 48106, (313)572-4334; 1989. This book was written to help professional and family caregivers better understand the various causes of behaviors such as wandering, resistance to care, incontinence and agitation. Problem-solving strategies for managing these behaviors are suggested. $13 (includes shipping); make checks payable to Eastern Michigan University.

Untie the Elderly, The Kendal Corporation, P.O. Box 100, Kennett Square, PA 19348. This newsletter on restraint reduction is available by writing and requesting to be placed on the mailing list.

Validation: The Feil Method, N. Feil, Edward Feil Productions, 4614 Prospect Avenue, Cleveland, OH 44103, (216)881-0040. This book provides information and ideas on how to interact with the disoriented resident. $10 (plus $2.50 shipping).

Wilfrid Gordon McDonald Partridge, M. Fox, Puffin Books, 1987. This illustrated children's book describes how a young boy helped an elderly resident find her memory. $7.95 or $13.95 hardcover.

VIDEOS

Before the Going Gets Rough (Part I), *After the Going Gets Rough* (Part II). Good Samaritan Hospital, Good Samaritan Family Support

Services, 1015 NW 22nd, Portland, Oregon 97210, (503)229-7348. These videos focus on the problem of aggressive behavior in persons with some form of confusion. Part I (30 min) presents ways to prevent and manage aggressive behavior. It identifies triggers, warning signs, and ways to diffuse and prevent problems. Part II (30 min) discusses the management of assaultive episodes. Sale (Part I or II) $250; rental (Part I or II) $65; sale (Parts I & II) $475; Rental (Parts I & II) $100. Includes manual.

Caring for Residents with Dementia, Benedictine Institute for Long Term Care, Mt. Angel, Oregon 97362, (503)845-9495, FAX (503)845-9210. 1/2" videocassette, 51 minutes/color, 1992. This video presents an overview of dementia, including important concepts such as excess disability, catastrophic reactions, agenda behavior, and verbal and nonverbal communication techniques. It suggests a problem-solving framework for addressing behavioral symptoms that energizes staff and fosters creativity. Study material, discussion questions and bibliography is available with tape. One week rental $40 plus $5 shipping and handling.

Caring for the Alzheimer's Resident: A Day in the Life of Nancy Moore, The Duke Family Support Program, Center for Study of Aging and Human Development, P.O. Box 3600, Duke University Medical Center, Durham, NC 27710, (919)660-7510. This video is an inexpensive tool that demonstrates the critical role of the nurse's aide in dealing with difficult behaviors. Cost $25 (postage and handling included).

Choice Among Risks: Physical Restraints Rejected, Health Professions Press, PO Box 10624, Baltimore, MD 10624, (401)337-9585. A useful tool for educating staff and helping to change attitudes. Length 30 minutes. Cost $70 to purchase; $35 preview charge (may have for 10 days).

The Corinne Dolan Alzheimer Center book and videotape package, C.D.A.C. at Heather Hill, 12340 Bass Lake Road, Chardon, OH 44024. The Corinne Dolan Alzheimer Center at Heather Hill presents an alternative approach to the care of persons with Alzheimer's disease. The book provides descriptions of the

Center's services, program activities, admissions criteria and process, staff duties and training, and research activities. The videotape focuses on the architectural features and provides an opportunity to experience the interaction of program and design. $20 (U.S. orders), $26 (Canadian orders), and $36 (overseas orders), price includes shipping and handling. Make checks payable to Dissemination Package.

Creative Interventions with the Alzheimer's Patient, Geriatric Resources, 931 S. Semoran Blvd., #200, Winter Park, FL 32792; (407)678-1616, FAX (407)678-5925. This three-tape series, by Mary Lucero, a well-known expert on care of persons with dementia, is designed to provide an introduction into understanding behavioral symptoms associated with Alzheimer's disease, current functional assessment tools, and interventions for proper caregiving. It comes with a 35-page handout. Three tapes and handout, is $340 (plus $5 for shipping).

Designing the Physical Environment for Persons with Dementia, Terra Nova Films, Inc., 9848 S. Winchester Avenue, Chicago, Illinois 60643, (312)881-8491. 1/2" videocassette and slides/20 min/ color/1987. Producer: D. Coons. Describes Wesley Hall, a special care unit for persons with dementia. Examples of activities, attitudes, and homelike environment helpful for persons with dementia. Sale, $110 (video); $175 (slides); rental, $45 (video only).

Looking for Yesterday, Edward Feil Productions, 4614 Prospect Avenue, Cleveland, Ohio 44103, (216)881-0040. 29 minutes; video shows how Validation Therapy offers hope to disoriented residents and staff caring for them. Sale, $335 (plus $5 shipping); rental: 1-day use, $25 (plus $7 shipping); 5-day use, $50 plus $7 shipping).

Managing & Understanding Behavior Problems in Alzheimer's Disease and Related Disorders, Northwest Geriatric Education Center, University of Washington, HL-23 Seattle, WA 98195, (206)685-7478. This 10-module videotape series includes 10 videotapes and a written manual. It is a training program geared for institutional staff, covering an overview of dementia, depression, delirium, and managing behaviors such as aggression, hallucinations, wandering, and inappropriate sexual behaviors. A promotional videotape is available for preview. Module series and manual, $250. Make checks payable to University of Washington/Alzheimer's Videos.

PEEGE, Phoenix/BFA Films & Video, 2349 Chaffee Dr., St. Louis, MO 63146, (314)569-0211. 28-minute/color/16 mm/1976. Producers: D. Knapp and L. Berman. Shows a family's painful visit to a nursing home to see their mother and grandmother, who is demented. A moving tape that illustrates the importance of connecting and communicating through reminiscence. The tape also deals with loss and grief. A good way to sensitize staff to their own losses and to help them see demented residents as whole people. $325 (plus $8.25 shipping).

Retrain Don't Restrain, American Association of Homes for the Aging, (mail orders) AAHA Publication, Dept. 5117, Washington, DC 20061-5117. Phone orders prepaid (VISA/Mastercard) AAHA Publication, 341 Victory Drive, Herndon, VA 20070. Available also through American Health Care Association, PO Box 96906, Washington, DC 20090-6906, 1(800)321-0343. This video illustrates the interdisciplinary process of restraint reduction and includes a variety of alternatives. Developed through the New York Jewish Home Hospital for the Aged, Restraint Minimization Project. $99 if facility is a member of either AAHA or AHCA; $129 if not. Price includes video, trainer's manual, and 10 workbooks; shipping for either, $13.

Wesley Hall: A Special Life, Terra Nova Films, Inc., 9848 S Winchester Avenue, Chicago, Illinois 60643, (312)881-8491. 16 mm, 1/2" and 3/4" videocassette/28 min/color/1986. Producer: Institute of Gerontology, University of Michigan. The film is about a special unit designed for persons with dementia. It presents visual attitudes, environment, and approaches that are helpful. Sale $245 (video); rental $55 (plus $7 shipping).

Working with the Confused Elderly Clients, Benedictine Institute for Long Term Care, 540 South Main Street, Mt. Angel, Oregon 97362, (503)845-9495, FAX (503)845-9210. 1/2" and 3/4" videocassette, 29 min/color/1986. This video teaches specific verbal and nonverbal communication techniques designed to increase staff skills and decrease behaviors such as wandering and agitation often associated with dementia. Sale, $200 (plus $5 shipping); rental (7-days) $35 (plus $5 shipping).

ACTIVITIES

Cross Creek Recreational Products, P.O. Box 289, Millbrook, NY 12545, (800)645-5816. Toys and devices for people to hold and manipulate, including the Tangle. Call for information and cost.

Eldergames, 11710 Hunters Lane, Rockville, MD 20852, (301)984-8336, (800)637-2604. Company makes products designed to stimulate memory and thought for persons with dementia. Games called Eldertrivia, Memory Joggers, Feel & Fold. Cost varies.

Geriatric Resources, Inc., 931 Semoran Blvd. #200, Winterpark, FL 32792, (407)678-1616. Sensory stimulation products for persons with dementia. Cost varies with product.

Songs to Remember, Hearth Song Productions, PO Box 211, Mt. Angel, Oregon 97362. This is a series of cassette tapes specifically developed for the older population. Tapes 1–3 contain songs for the Catholic, Protestant, and contemporary Christian traditions, respectively. Tape 4 contains old popular favorites. Set of 4 is $39 (shipping and handling $3); individual tapes are $10 (shipping and handling $1.50).

Susquehanna Rehab Products, Road 2, Box 41, 9 Overlook Drive, Wrightsville, PA 17368, (800)248-2011. Includes Fiddle link, wrist-a-twist for people to hold and manipulate, as well as Footstool. Call for information and cost.

POSITIONING DEVICES

Adirondak Chairs (Estate Chairs), Manufactured by Rubbermaid. Available from outdoor furniture stores.

Cheese Leaner Cushion, Clock Medical Supply, 118–124 East 9th, Winfield, KN 67156, (800)527-0049. This cushion is used to prevent lateral slumping in wheelchairs, recliners, and gerichairs. $24.95 with cotton cover; $31.95 with naugahyde. UPS plus $1.50 handling.

Dycem, Alimed, 297 High Street, Dedham, MA 02026, (617)329-2900, FAX (617)329-8392. A nonslip, rubberlike plastic material that is placed in the chair seat to prevent sliding (16 in. × 2 yds.) #8273. $34.95. Also available in many sizes and configurations. (Can be obtained from many health equipment companies.)

Foam Elevating Inserts (for use with trough BK-6462-01, Fred Sammons, P.O. Box 32, Brookfield, IL 60513, (800)323-5547, FAX (800)547-4333. Call for information and cost.

Inflatable Seat Cushions, Roho, P.O. Box 658, Belleville, IL 62222, (800)851-3449, FAX (618)277-6518. Call for information and cost.

LiteNest, Orthopedic Products Corporation, 10381 W. Jefferson Blvd., Culver City, CA, (800)432-2225. This ultralight portable system weighs less than 4 pounds. It also incorporates an integrated seat and back design with a mutidensity foam pad. $199; an incontinence cover is available for slightly more.

Seats, Cushions & Backs, Jay Medical, Ltd., P.O. Box 18656, Boulder, CO, 83038-8656, (800)648-8282. Call for information and cost.

Skil-Care, 167 Saw Mill River Road, Yonkers, NY 10701, (800)431-2972. This company has developed a group of products called PASS (Patient Autonomy Safety Systems). They include self-release devices and positioning cushions. A video is available at no cost on a 30-day loaner basis.

Sit-Straight Cushion, AliMed, Inc., 297 High Street, Dedham, MA 02026, (617)329-2900, FAX (617)329-8392. Two sizes are available, 16 × 18 inches (product #1250) and 16 × 16 inches (product #1251). $39.95 each.

Solid Seat Inserts, AliMed, 297 High Street, Dedham, MA 02026, (617)329-2900, FAX (617)329-8392. This wheelchair insert eliminates the discomfort caused by sling seats. It creates a flat, stable seating surface. Also comes in wedge shape. The inserts (uncovered) are available in two sizes 16 × 18 inches (product #1192) and 16 × 16 inches (product #1193). $24 each; also offered covered for $35 each.

Super Constructa Foam, AliMed, 297 High Street, Dedham, MA 02026, (617)329-2900, FAX (617)329-8392. This dense, closed cell foam can be easily cut to form custom-made positioning wedges and supports. Call for price and information.

Ultra-Form Wedge Cushion, American Health Systems, Inc., P.O. Box 26688, Greenville, SC 29616-1688. Call (800)234-6655 for the number of your local representative who will quote you a price). This wedge-shaped chair cushion prevents sliding in addition to providing pressure relief. $91.60 (case of 4 without covers), Protect cover $30 each; Durable cover $34.90 each. Shipping and handling will vary.

Varilite Chair Cushion, Cascade Designs, Inc., 4000 1st Ave. S., Seattle, WA 98134, (800)527-1527 FAX (206)467-9421. This lightweight chair cushion/seating system can have a firm or soft base with two to four self-inflating modular cushions that compensate precisely for posture deviation. $250–$310 depending on the number of cushions selected.

WheelNest, Orthopedic Products Corporation, 10381 W. Jefferson Blvd., Culver City, CA 90232, (800)432-3335. This is a portable, easy-to-install integrated seating system incorporating Akton™ solid polymer. It provides a solid seat and back support and requires no maintenance. It has an available incontinence cover with nonslip base and components to enhance its positioning. $319.

BARRIERS

Door Guard: Vinyl Barrier, Bussard & Son, Inc. Custom Canvassing, 425 SW Jackson Street, Albany, OR 97321, (503)926-7747. A vinyl barrier for wanderers (yellow strip). This visual barrier meets fire code standards and can prevent problems with wanderers. $10 plus UPS; 60" × 480". Price may vary according to size.

Stopper Kit, Clock Medical, P.O. Box 620, Winfield, KS 67156, (800)527-0049. Includes "stop" signs, "do not enter" signs, and mesh strips to put across doors. Call for information and cost.

MOBILITY EQUIPMENT

Able Walker, Brandt Enterprises, P.O. Box 491, Donald, OR 97020, (800)426-6857. A four-wheeled walker with brakes and shopping basket that converts to a seat. $349.

Armrest (padded flipaway), Therafin Corporation, 19747 Wolf Road, Mokena, IL 60448, (708)479-7300, FAX (708)479-1515; order line, (800)843-7234. $144.95; call for a representative in your area.

Carolina Rocker, ARTEC, Inc., Health Products, P.O. Box 25103, Greenville, SC 29616, (803)288-2111 or (800)445-0234. Converts a wheelchair into a rocker. Good for agitation, restlessness, tardive dyskinesia movements. For price call Flaghouse, (800)221-5185 or Geriatric Resources, (407)678-1616.

Chariot Ambulator, First Choice International, 12 Westerville Square #335, Westerville, OH 43081, (800)235-0370. This is an adult walking frame for residents with good trunk balance who stand or walk unsteadily. $495 in the continental U.S. plus $38.50 shipping and handling.

Drop Seats (hardware), Adaptive Engineering Lab, Inc., 4403 Russell Road 2S-3, Mukilteo, WA 98275-5018, (800)327-6080. Call for information and cost.

Forearm Walker and Attachment, Legacy Medical, 6040 N. Cutter Circle, #309, Portland, OR 97217, (503)289-9314. This walker has a horseshoe-shaped upholstered forearm support and adjustable hand grips. Allows individuals to walk more upright than with traditional walkers and provides increased sense of support and comfort. $148 walker with wheels; $209 platform attachment. Shipping and handling included.

Go-Chair, Canhart Industries Ltd., 140 Renfrew Dr., Suite 205, Markham, Ontario, Canada, L3R 6B3, (800)265-7400. This wheelchair comes in a variety of models. It is attractive, easy to turn and manipulate, and nontippable; promotes independent wheelchair mobility. $1,000+ (varies with model).

Ultimate Walker (formerly Merry Walker), Direct Supply, 6761 N. Industrial Road, Milwaukee, WI 53223, (800)634-7328. This adjustible wheeled walking frame (made from PVC pipe) allows residents to walk or wheel seated or standing. It is useful for residents who stand unsteadily or are unsafely mobile on their own. Cost is approximately $300.00 plus shipping and handling. (Price varies according to quantity.)

Life-Ride Chair, Arjo-Century, 6380 Oakton Street, Morton Grove, IL 60053, (800)323-1245, FAX (708)967-1241. This life has a sling seat and/or a spade seat that allows one person to transfer individuals without manual lifting. Also can convert to a walker for ambulation training. Approximately $2,900.

Next Step & Rover, Noble Motion, Inc., P.O. Box 5366, 5871 Center Avenue, Pittsburgh, PA 15206, (800)234-9255. These are four-wheeled 8-inch solid-tire walkers with hand brakes. Additional accessories can also be purchased. Available in single hand brake model. Cost $375–$450 (free delivery).

Posture-Guard Wheeled Recliner, May Corp. and Step-Saver, Inc., call (800)525-3590. This tilt-in-space wheeled recliner with independently operated leg rests is useful for residents who are severely impaired and slide or lean in regular wheelchairs and recliners. Cost starts around $455 and varies with options and models. For information or a free demonstration call the above number.

Scoot Gard, This nonskid matting is used for boats and RV's. Can be used in place of Dycem. It is washable and has anti-microbial properities to inhibit bacteria and mildew. Can be purchased at many stores. Cost $.79/foot or $8.99 for 1 × 12 foot roll.

Tilt-in-Space Wheelchair, Lumex, 100 Spence Street, Bay Shore, NY 11706-2290, (800)645-5272. Call for a representative in your area.

PRESSURE CHANGE ALARMS

Pressure change alarms for beds and chairs—These devices have a sensor pad that goes under the mattress or chair seat that sets off an alarm when the resident tries to leave. Some can be adapted for wheelchairs. They have an advantage over the position change alarms because the resident cannot remove them.

Bed-Check, Bed-Check, 4408 S. Harvard #A, Tulsa, OK 74135, (800)523-7956.

Code Alert, RF Technologies, Inc., 3720 North 124th Street, Milwaukie, WI 53222, (800)669-9946, FAX (414)466-1806.

Posey Sitter, Posey Company, 5635 Peck Road, Arcadia, CA 91006-0020, (800)44-POSEY or (818)443-3143.

POSITION CHANGE ALARMS

These alarms alert staff when a resident changes position, such as going from a seated to a standing position. This is done in a variety of ways, such as a sensor or a cord-like tether.

Ambularm, Alert Care Inc., Shelter Point Business Center, 591 Redwood Hwy., Suite 2125, Mill Valley, CA 94941, (800)826-7444. Approximate price $170. The Ambularm is a lightweight, position sensitive alarm worn on the thigh.

Chair Sentinel, Powderhorn Industries, 931 N. Park Ave., PO Box 1443, Montrose, CO 81402. This is a resident releasable wheelchair seatbelt that emits an alarm when unfastened. Cost $150.

Mugger Stopper, Safety Technology International, Inc., 2306 Airport Road., Waterford, MI 48327, (313)673-9898 or (800)888-4784. This device has to be adapted before it can serve as a position change alarm. The advantage is cost. Cost approximately $15.

TABS™ Mobility Monitor, WanderGuard, Inc., 941 "O" Street, Suite 205, Lincoln, NE 68501, (800)824-2996, FAX (402)475-4281.

Window/Door Alarm, Radio Shack (check phone directory for your local outlet). This device has to be adapted to function as a position change alarm. Cost approximately $15.

EXIT ALARMS

Baby Nursery Monitors, Fisher Price and Others. These devices allow you to hear if someone is moving about or calling out.
Alert Care Exit Alarm (see Ambularm).

TRACKING

Care Trak, Wildlife Materials, Inc., Route 1, Box 427A, Carbondale, IL 62901, (800)842-4537. A radio tracking system that sounds an alarm when a wanderer leaves monitored areas; a mobile locator helps staff find the resident. Cost varies from $810 to $4,310 depending on several variables. Call for cost.

SIMULATION: A METHOD TO UNDERSTAND PHYSICAL CHANGES ASSOCIATED WITH AGING

by Vicki L. Schmall, PhD
Oregon State University,
Extension Gerontology Specialist

A method to help people understand the physical changes associated with aging is simulated activities. Individuals are given "handicapping" conditions that approximate reality and are required to complete common day-to-day tasks.

METHODS/MATERIALS

Sight

With increasing age, the eyes decrease in their ability to see clearly, particularly small details such as the eye of a needle or directions on medication containers. The average 65-year-old has visual acuity of 20/70 or less. Several studies suggest that the lens of the eye yellows with age and filters out colors at the blue end of the light spectrum. Warm colors (yellow, orange, and red) are more easily distinguished by many older people than cool colors (blue, green, and violet).

To partially impair vision, fold cellophane or plastic wrap several times and place over eyes or glasses. Yellow cellophane is recommended. Cheesecloth, gauze, sunglasses or laboratory protective glasses smeared with petroleum jelly also are effective.

Loss of peripheral vision, as caused by glaucoma, can be simulated by covering the temple area and lenses of glass frames with nontransparent contact paper, leaving a 1/4-inch diameter hole in the center of each lens. Loss of central vision, as occurs in macular degeneration, can be simulated by covering the inner half of the lenses of glasses with contact paper.

Hearing

Two major hearing losses that occur with age are (1) presbycusis—loss in the ability to hear high-frequency sounds; and (2) decibel loss—reduced ability to hear sounds of low intensity.

Industrial earplugs are most effective for simulating volume loss. Alternative methods include using cotton balls or swimmer earplugs or playing an audiotape, television, or radio at a low sound level. A more pronounced effect can be obtained by wearing earmuffs or stereo headphones.

Several media simulate hearing and/or vision changes common in the later years. These include a cassette audiotape "Challenging Listening Situations for Older People," $20, and a slide tape program, "Age-Related Vision and Hearing Changes," $95. Both are available from University of Michigan Medical Center, Media Library, R 4440 Kresge 3, Ann Arbor, MI 48109-0518).

Taste

Food that smells and tastes good is important to good nutrition. Many older people, however, experience a decline in their ability to taste and smell. A common complaint of the very old is that "the food just doesn't taste good anymore" or "this food tastes sour or bitter."

Foods that are bland or saltless—for example, saltless crackers and colored water, unsweetened drink mix, or weak lemonade—

can be used to simulate loss of taste sensitivity. A recipe for "tasteless cookies" follows: Sift together 2 cups flour and 1/2 teaspoon baking powder. Blend in 1/2 cup shortening. Add 2 eggs. Refrigerate 1 hour. Roll into small balls and press flat with the tines of a fork. Bake at 400°, 6–8 minutes. Makes approximately 60 cookies, about 1 inch in diameter.

Smell

To simulate loss in the ability to smell, use nose plugs, place cotton in the nose, or hold the nostrils closed. Blindfold individuals and present them with a variety of odors to identify.

Touch

Skin sensitivity and the ability to detect pain decreases with age. Older persons distinguish textures by touch alone. Because pain threshold increases, an older person is more apt to be cut or burned and not know it until severe damage has occurred. For example, the hot temperature of bath water or a heating pad may not be felt readily.

Loss of tactile sensitivity may be simulated by wearing latex or surgical gloves, wrapping tape around the tips of fingers, or applying rubber cement to the fingertips and letting it dry.

Mobility/Dexterity

Bone and muscular changes mean decreased ability to ambulate and slowness in movement for some older people. Illnesses such as arthritis, Parkinson's disease, and stroke may severely limit a person's dexterity or mobility.

To simulate loss of finger dexterity, wrap masking tape around each finger, particularly the thumb and index finger, or tape splints on several fingers. Knee and elbow joints may be immobilized by using splints or wrapping them with 3- or 4-inch elastic bandages. Have individuals also use a wheelchair, cane, crutches, or walker.

More than one impairment may be experienced simultaneously to simulate multiple physical limitations. For example, a person may be made both vision- and hearing-impaired.

ACTIVITIES

Give the "impaired" several tasks. The visually impaired might be asked to find a number in the telephone directory, prepare a meal, read an article in the newspaper, or thread a needle. The blind person might be asked to peel a cucumber or eat a meal. An "arthritic" individual might be asked to open a child-proof container and perform such everyday tasks as tying shoelaces, peeling an orange, buttoning a shirt, or writing a letter.

Utilize everyday activities that the nonhandicapped often take for granted but which may be more difficult or take more time to accomplish by the person who has a physical impairment. By limiting the time to complete tasks, individuals will experience the frustration that persons who have physical limitations sometimes feel when others unduly hasten them.

DISCUSSION

Following the simulated activities discuss participants' reactions and feelings. Focus on implications of impairments for older adults and for workshop participants as they work and relate to older persons who have physical impairments. Emphasize that most older people are in relatively good health, and for those older persons who experience such physical changes, many compensate for them in various ways.

RESOURCES

Two publications of the Oregon State University Extension Service are helpful in conducting programs on sensory changes and aging:

- PNW 196, *Sensory Changes in Later Life*
  Discusses the sensory changes—vision, hearing, taste, smell, and touch that commonly occur in later life and the implications of these changes for the older person and for those who work with elders. Order from Publication Orders, Agricultural Communications, Oregon State University, Administrative Services Building 422, Corvallis, OR 97331-2119, (503)737-2513. Single copies, $1.00 plus $.50 for postage.
- A comprehensive teaching guide, HE 12-001L, *Growing Older: Sensory Changes*, is available for $1.25 from Extension Gerontology, Oregon State University, Milam Hall 161, Corvallis, OR 97331-5106; (503)737-1014.

Used with permission from Oregon State University Extension Service—SP 54-077. Revised January 1992.

INDEX

Abstraction activity interventions, 202
Activity interventions
  carpenter's role in
    miscellaneous activities and, 205–206
    music and, 204
    physical activity and, 205
    reminiscence and, 204–205
    storytelling and, 204
    types of activities and, 203–204
  conclusions regarding, 206
  detective's role in, 200–201
    abstraction and, 202
    emotional needs and, 202
    judgment and, 202
    language and, 202
    memory and, 201
    organization of movement and, 201
    perception dysfunction and, 201
  importance of, 197–198
  levels of, 69
  magician's role in
    experiential exercises and, 198–199
    understanding the resident and, 199–200
  psychosocial environment and, 75–76
  resource list of, 276
  See also Psychosocial, activity interventions
Administration. See Organizational environment
Advance directives, 11
Agency for Health Care Policy

Research (AHCPR), 214
Agenda behavior, 193–195
Aggressive behavior. See Problematic behavior
Aging process
  drug therapy and, 210–211
  simulation exercises of, 283–287
Agnosia, 201
Alprazolam, 215, 264, 265
Alzheimer's Association, 255
American Association of Homes for the Aging, 255
American Health Care Association, 255
Amitriptyline, 215, 263
Amoxapine, 263
Antianxiety drugs
  benzodiazepines as, 215
  guidelines for use of, 216
  indications for, 216
  See also Anxiolytic drugs; specific drug name
Antidepressant medication
  adverse effects of, 214
  bereavement, self-esteem and, 41–42
  commonly used examples of, 263
  diagnoses pertinent to use of, 261
  major depression symptoms and, 261–262
  older vs. newer agents of, 214–215
  side effects of, 262–263
  terminology regarding, 213
  use guidelines for, 214
  use, misuse of, 214
  See also specific drug name
Antimanic drugs, 218–219